# Skin Allergy

*Editor*

SUSAN NEDOROST

# IMMUNOLOGY AND ALLERGY CLINICS OF NORTH AMERICA

www.immunology.theclinics.com

August 2021 • Volume 41 • Number 3

**ELSEVIER**

1600 John F. Kennedy Boulevard • Suite 1800 • Philadelphia, Pennsylvania, 19103-2899

http://www.theclinics.com

**IMMUNOLOGY AND ALLERGY CLINICS OF NORTH AMERICA Volume 41, Number 3**

**August 2021 ISSN 0889-8561, ISBN-13: 978-0-323-81345-7**

Editor: Katerina Heidhausen

Developmental Editor: Jessica Cañaberal

*Immunology and Allergy Clinics of North America* (ISSN 0889–8561) is published quarterly by Elsevier Inc., 360 Park Avenue South, New York, NY 10010-1710. Months of issue are February, May, August, and November. Periodicals postage paid at New York, NY and additional mailing offices. Subscription prices are $347.00 per year for US individuals, $827.00 per year for US institutions, $100.00 per year for US students and residents, $423.00 per year for Canadian individuals, $100.00 per year for Canadian students, $864.00 per year for Canadian institutions, $447.00 per year for international individuals, $864.00 per year for international institutions, $220.00 per year for international students. To receive student/resident rate, orders must be accompanied by name of affiliated institution, date of term, and the *signature* of program/residency coordinator on institution letterhead. Orders will be billed at individual rate until proof of status is received. Foreign air speed delivery is included in all *Clinics* subscription prices. All prices are subject to change without notice. **POSTMASTER:** Send address changes to *Immunology and Allergy Clinics of North America,* Elsevier Health Sciences Division, Subscription Customer Service, 3251 Riverport Lane, Maryland Heights, MO 63043. **Customer Service: 1-800-654-2452 (U.S. and Canada); 314-447-8871 (outside U.S. and Canada). Fax: 314-447-8029. E-mail: journalscustomerservice-usa@elsevier.com (for print support); journalsonlinesupport-usa@elsevier.com (for online support).**

*Reprints.* For copies of 100 or more, of articles in this publication, please contact the Commercial Reprints Department, Elsevier Inc., 360 Park Avenue South, New York, New York 10010-1710. Tel. 212-633-3874, Fax: 212-633-3820, E-mail: reprints@elsevier.com.

*Immunology and Allergy Clinics of North America is covered in MEDLINE/PubMed (Index Medicus), Current Contents/Life Sciences, Science Citation Index, ISI/BIOMED, Chemical Abstracts, and EMBASE/Excerpta Medica.*

# Contributors

## EDITOR

**SUSAN NEDOROST, MD**
Professor, Dermatology and Population and Quantitative Health Sciences, University Hospitals Cleveland Medical Center/Case Western Reserve University, Cleveland, Ohio, USA

## AUTHORS

**MARY KATHRYN ABEL, AB**
Department of Dermatology, University of California, San Francisco, UCSF School of Medicine, San Francisco, California, USA

**DAMIEN ABREU, MD, PhD**
Medical Scientist Training Program, Division of Dermatology, Department of Medicine, Washington University School of Medicine, St Louis, Missouri, USA

**STACEY E. ANDERSON, PhD**
Health Effects Laboratory Division, National Institute for Occupational Safety and Health, Morgantown, West Virginia, USA

**ALYSSA GWEN ASHBAUGH, MD**
Department of Dermatology, University of California, San Francisco, San Francisco, California, USA; School of Medicine, University of California, Irvine, Irvine, California, USA

**MOHSEN BAGHCHECHI, BS**
University of California, Riverside, School of Medicine, Riverside, California, USA

**OKSANA A. BAILIFF, MD**
Dermatology Resident PGY-4, Geisinger Medical Center, Danville, Pennsylvania, USA

**SARA BILIMORIA, MS**
Northwestern University Feinberg School of Medicine, Chicago, Illinois, USA

**KANWALJIT K. BRAR, MD**
Assistant Professor, Department of Pediatrics, NYU Grossman School of Medicine, Hassenfeld Children's Hospital, New York, New York, USA

**CHRISTEN BROWN, BS**
Tulane University School of Medicine, New Orleans, Louisiana, USA

**JENNIFER K. CHEN, MD**
Clinical Associate Professor, Department of Dermatology, Stanford University School of Medicine, Redwood City, California, USA

**ITAI CHIPINDA, PhD**
Global Product Stewardship & Toxicology, Bartlesville, Oklahoma, USA

**ELISE FOURNIER, BS**
Michigan State University, East Lansing, Michigan, USA

**ANA M. GIMENEZ-ARNAU, MD**
Department of Dermatology, Hospital del Mar, Universitat Autònoma de Barcelona, Barcelona, Spain

**ALINA GOLDENBERG, MD, MAS**
Dermatologist Medical Group of North County, San Diego, California, USA

**DOROTHY LINN HOLNESS, MD, MHSc, DTS, FRCPC, FFOM(Hon)**
Professor Emerita, Department of Medicine and Dalla Lana School of Public Health, University of Toronto, Staff Physician, Division of Occupational Medicine, Department of Medicine, Associate Scientist, MAP Centre for Urban Health Solutions, Li Ka Shing Knowledge Institute, St Michael's Hospital, Toronto, Ontario, Canada

**SHARON E. JACOB, MD**
Veterans Health Administration, Loma Linda, Dermatology Section Chief, Loma Linda, California, USA; Health Sciences Professor of Medicine and Pediatrics (Dermatology), University of California, Riverside, School of Medicine, Riverside, California, USA

**LILLY KERCHINSKY, BS**
Michigan State University, East Lansing, Michigan, USA

**BRIAN S. KIM, MD, MTR**
Associate Professor of Dermatology, Division of Dermatology, Department of Medicine, Center for the Study of Itch and Sensory Disorders, Department of Anesthesiology, Department of Pathology and Immunology, Washington University School of Medicine, St Louis, Missouri, USA

**PETER LIO, MD**
Clinical Assistant Professor of Dermatology and Pediatrics, Northwestern University Feinberg School of Medicine, Chicago, Illinois, USA

**HOWARD MAIBACH, MD**
Department of Dermatology, University of California, San Francisco, San Francisco, California, USA

**CHRISTEN M. MOWAD, MD**
Chair of the Division of Dermatology, Geisinger Medical Center, Danville, Pennsylvania, USA

**JENNY E. MURASE, MD**
Department of Dermatology, University of California, San Francisco, San Francisco, California, USA; Department of Dermatology, Palo Alto Foundation Medical Group, Mountain View, California, USA

**JANNETT NGUYEN, MD**
Resident, Department of Dermatology, Stanford University School of Medicine, Redwood City, California, USA

**ANDREW SCHEMAN, MD**
Professor of Clinical Dermatology, Northwestern University Feinberg School of Medicine, Chicago, Illinois, USA

**PAUL D. SIEGEL, PhD**
Health Effects Laboratory Division, National Institute for Occupational Safety and Health, Morgantown, West Virginia, USA

**KYLE TEGTMEYER, BS**
Northwestern University Feinberg School of Medicine, Chicago, Illinois, USA

**JASON WEI, BS**
University of Illinois Urbana-Champaign, Urbana, Illinois, USA

**JIADE YU, MD**
Department of Dermatology, Massachusetts General Hospital, Harvard Medical School, Boston, Massachusetts, USA

# Contents

of ACD. The Pediatric Baseline Series was recently published by expert consensus for use in pediatric patch testing, with additional allergens tested as guided by history. This article examines methods of patch testing and up-to-date data on pediatric ACD. The top allergens are reviewed, and avoidance strategies are discussed.

Allergic contact dermatitis (ACD) remains a globally prevalent disease for both children and adults. The silent ACD epidemic continues to be fueled by the introduction of novel allergens in industrial and household products and the continued presence of known allergens. In 1997, Allan Dillarstone noted a sinusoidal pattern to epidemics when allergenic preservatives were replaced by alternative chemicals within the market, which then similarly increased in allergenicity. A call for public health vigilance and prevention initiatives is needed to intervene in the ACD epidemic.

This article reviews the laboratory's role in identifying causes of chemical-induced allergic dermatitis. Several topics will be discussed. Allergen hazard identification refers to testing of chemicals for their sensitization potential. Animal-based, in silico, in chemico, and in vitro tests have been developed to identify the skin sensitization hazard of potential chemical allergens, but only a few of these are accepted by regulatory agencies. Laboratory investigations have also evaluated the stability of several commercially available allergic contact dermatitis patch tests. Such studies are considered product testing and are usually conducted in analytical chemistry laboratories.

Occupational contact dermatitis is the most common occupational skin disease (OSD), and most of them are irritant in nature. There is less information available about contact urticaria than contact dermatitis. There are several strategies to prevent OSD, although workplace studies suggest there are gaps in their use in the workplace. Because early detection leads to improved outcomes, screening for dermatitis in industries such as health care would be useful. Both diagnosis and management involve 2 components: the actual disease diagnosis and medical treatment and the work-relatedness and management of the workplace to reduce exposures.

Allergen avoidance is the most effective treatment of contact allergy. Patient improvement ultimately relies on identification of safe alternative products, which can be used by the patient. Safe personal care product options typically can be found using ingredient database programs. Avoidance of allergens in other products (eg, shoes, clothing, and dental care) often is challenging. This article discusses specific safe alternatives for the 80 allergens on the 2017 American Contact Dermatitis Society core allergen series.

This article discusses contact urticaria syndrome definition, history, epidemiology, occupational relevance, mechanisms, clinical manifestations, diagnostic tools, agents responsible, and how to prevent and treat the patients affected. Contact urticaria syndrome is often misdiagnosed because it is not well known or recognized by physicians. Commonly the patient recognizes the cause of the clinical symptom, but the cause can be exceptional or new. Triggers include proteins, chemical compounds, agricultural chemicals, metals, plants, foods, and other substances. The objective of this article is to help dermatologists, toxicologists, and immunologists by providing diagnostic tools to avoid the culprit agent and treat the patients.

Protein contact dermatitis is a cutaneous hypersensitivity reaction after chronic, recurrent exposure or chronic irritation to animal or plant protein. Although the pathophysiological mechanisms underlying protein contact dermatitis are not well characterized, protein contact dermatitis is thought to be caused by combined type I/IV-mediated, type-1 mediated, or a Langerhans cell immunoglobulin E–mediated delayed hypersensitivity reaction. This chapter reviews the epidemiology, pathogenesis, clinical features, common protein allergens, diagnostic process, treatment options, and prognosis of protein contact dermatitis.

Dermatitis is a common condition frequently encountered by dermatologists. The diagnosis of dermatitis can be challenging because this condition is often multifactorial, and many skin diseases that can mimic dermatitis should be considered in the differential diagnosis. It is important to recognize and be familiar with these conditions because some of them can represent signs of systemic disease or malignancies and misdiagnosis can lead to mismanagement and adverse outcomes for the patient.

Food allergy evaluation for dermatologic disorders is warranted when Type 1 allergy is suspected, and includes skin prick testing (SPT) or measurement of specific immunoglobulin E (IgE) levels. The utility of these tests for identifying triggers is improved with clinical correlation, especially for contact urticaria, and protein contact dermatitis, which are mixed mechanism diseases. In atopic dermatitis (AD), patients are at risk for development of food allergy, and screening with SPT or IgE may be considered in severe AD, especially to guide early food introduction. Management of food-related AD exacerbations should focus on modifications in skincare before evaluating for allergy.

x

*Skin Allergy*

# IMMUNOLOGY AND ALLERGY CLINICS OF NORTH AMERICA

---

### SERIES OF RELATED INTEREST

*Medical Clinics*
https://www.medical.theclinics.com/

---

**THE CLINICS ARE AVAILABLE ONLINE!**
Access your subscription at:
www.theclinics.com

# Preface

# Modification of the Personal Environment as Treatment: Irritant and Allergic Dermatitis and Contact Urticaria

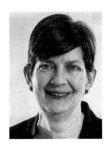

Susan Nedorost, MD
*Editor*

"Skin Allergy" is a plain language term that is patient-centric. Patients with dermatitis may suffer tremendous personal and occupational burden; they often question the role of environmental allergens as a cause of their symptoms. Our answers are complicated! The labels of atopic dermatitis, allergic contact dermatitis, and contact urticaria are not terribly useful to patients when they try to understand the role of allergy in their symptoms. This issue intentionally avoids the use of the terms "atopic" and "allergic contact" dermatitis in article titles, as these entities frequently overlap.

I often explain to patients that "there is no good treatment for the symptom of itch," and we have to treat the underlying skin disease. Abreu and Kim explain much about the mechanism of itch in their article in this issue! The "underlying neuroimmune crosstalk" between skin allergy and nerve cells has provided some potential new therapeutic targets, including MRGPRB2/X2-mast cell signaling axis in contact dermatitis. Lio and colleagues outline the complexity of mechanisms in skin allergy and emerging therapeutic targets.

Nguyen and Chen describe how distribution of dermatitis can provide clues to environmental causes. This can help guide selections of allergens for patch testing. Brown and Yu discuss patch testing in children, as we now recognize that allergic contact dermatitis occurs frequently in children both with and without atopic dermatitis.

Patch testing allows personalized avoidance strategies for allergic contact dermatitis. We need to be clear that allergens are not something we can, or should, eliminate from the planet in most cases. Jacob-Soo reviews epidemics of allergic contact dermatitis. Identification of the allergen causing an epidemic is often followed by

Immunol Allergy Clin N Am 41 (2021) xi–xiii
https://doi.org/10.1016/j.iac.2021.05.002
0889-8561/21/© 2021 Published by Elsevier Inc.

introduction of an alternative to replace the offending allergen, which often also turns out to be a contact allergen (the Dillarstone effect). Siegel and colleagues describe the difficulty in identifying new contact allergens and the laboratory techniques that can help.

Occupational skin disease requires great depth of knowledge due to the unique exposures in many occupations. Holness explains data collection on occupational dermatology diagnoses and reviews literature on impact (function and cost) of occupational skin disease. She summarizes benefits of screening, given that other preventive measures, for example, skin care with emollients, have not been shown to be helpful. This is likely because dermatitis is multifactorial, and emollients do not help all patients with dermatitis.[1]

*When allergic contact dermatitis occurs in healthy skin*, avoidance of identified allergens can be curative. Allergic Contact Dermatitis, with focus on conventional patch testing, was the subject of the July 2020 *Dermatologic Clinics*. Scheman and colleagues update us on alternative products to help our patients with allergic contact dermatitis to "conventional," nonprotein, contact allergens.

*When environmental allergies develop in chronically inflamed skin due to genetic barrier dysfunction ("atopic dermatitis") or wet work,* potential allergens expand to include those that are less common in the general population, such as proteins in food and commensal organisms. The immune response may be Th2 skewed and involve both delayed and immediate-type hypersensitivity. Gimenez-Arnau and Maibach discuss the many causes of contact urticaria. Murase and colleagues detail the many causes of protein contact dermatitis and urticaria.

Mowad and Bailiff discuss mimics of dermatitis. Knowledge of these mimics makes dermatologists a critical member of the health care team for patients with dermatitis. Brar explains the expertise that allergists can offer for patients at risk for immediate-type hypersensitivity. We now recognize that immediate-type hypersensitivity begins with percutaneous sensitization in most cases.

We still lack a reliable test to detect protein (eg, food or microbial) triggers for dermatitis. Skin prick tests are not specific for protein contact dermatitis. Atopy (protein) patch tests would be expected to be more specific[2] but are not yet standardized. Dr Brar reminds us that food avoidance may contribute to risk of immediate-type hypersensitivity with reintroduction of the food. Allergists can help us assess this risk.

Dermatitis truly is complicated! The mechanisms of allergy are complex, as is the connection to itch. Much dogma is at least partially wrong, including direction to all patients to apply moisturizers, to take antihistamines for itch, and to ignore the potential contribution of ingested foods or food additives to dermatitis.

I hope that this issue will broaden our collective thinking and better connect with our patients who suffer compromise of work and quality of life as a result of skin allergy.

Susan Nedorost, MD
Professor, Dermatology and Population and
Quantitative Health Sciences
University Hospitals Cleveland Medical Center/
Case Western Reserve University
11100 Euclid Avenue
Cleveland, OH 44106, USA

*E-mail address:*
stn@case.edu

**REFERENCES**

1. Leshem YA, Wong A, McClanahan D, et al. The effects of common over-the-counter moisturizers on skin barrier function: a randomized, observer-blind, within-patient, controlled study. Dermatitis 2020;31(5):309–15.
2. Pootongkam S, Havele SA, Orillaza H, et al. Atopy patch tests may identify patients at risk for systemic contact dermatitis. Immun Inflamm Dis 2020;8(1):24–9.

# Innate Immune Regulation of Dermatitis

Damien Abreu, MD, PhD[a,b], Brian S. Kim, MD, MTR[b,c,d,e],*

## KEYWORDS

- Atopic dermatitis (AD) • Allergic contact dermatitis (ACD) • Urticaria • Mast cells
- Mas-related G protein–coupled receptor (MRGPR) • Itch • Janus kinase (JAK)

## KEY POINTS

- Type 2 cytokine blockade and Janus kinase inhibition represent major advances in therapy for inflammatory skin disorders such as atopic dermatitis.
- New understanding of innate immunity is informing the pathophysiology of atopic dermatitis, allergic contact dermatitis, and chronic spontaneous urticaria.
- Newly recognized pathways such as the Mas-related G protein–coupled receptor B2 and Mas-related G protein–coupled receptor X2 receptors implicate mast cells in a variety of pruritic skin disorders such as allergic contact dermatitis, chronic spontaneous urticaria, and contact urticaria.

## INTRODUCTION

The skin is a dynamic organ comprised of a diverse network of epithelial, immune, and neuronal cells that integrate a variety of signals to provide a protective barrier, immunity, and sensation toward environmental insults. However, in the context of chronic inflammation, many of these homeostatic processes become dysregulated, resulting in pathologic outcomes such as the itch-scratch cycle, which can then be difficult to therapeutically disrupt. Recent advances in skin immunology have revealed new innate immune and neuroimmune mechanisms that are actively changing conventional paradigms of the pathophysiology underlying various inflammatory skin disorders. This article uses major discoveries in atopic dermatitis

[a] Medical Scientist Training Program, Washington University School of Medicine, Box 8226, 660 South Euclid Avenue, St. Louis, MO 63110-1093, USA; [b] Division of Dermatology, Department of Medicine, Washington University School of Medicine, St Louis, MO 63110, USA; [c] Center for the Study of Itch and Sensory Disorders, Washington University School of Medicine, St Louis, MO 63110, USA; [d] Department of Anesthesiology, Washington University School of Medicine, St Louis, MO 63110, USA; [e] Department of Pathology and Immunology, Washington University School of Medicine, St Louis, MO 63110, USA
* Corresponding author. 660 South Euclid Avenue, Campus Box 8123, St Louis, MO 63110.
E-mail address: briankim@wustl.edu
Twitter: @itchdoctor (B.S.K.)

Immunol Allergy Clin N Am 41 (2021) 347–359
https://doi.org/10.1016/j.iac.2021.04.011      immunology.theclinics.com

(AD), allergic contact dermatitis (ACD), and urticaria to highlight how the evolving understanding of skin immunology informs new therapeutic landscapes.

## THE SKIN IMMUNE NETWORK

Cutaneous immunity is orchestrated by a complex array of innate and adaptive immune cells residing across the various layers of the skin. The innate immune system responds briskly to nonspecific stimuli such as pathogen-associated molecular pattern motifs and epithelial cell-derived cytokines. Key innate effector cells include macrophages, basophils, mast cells, and innate lymphoid cells (ILCs). In contrast, the adaptive immune system can generate highly specific receptors on T cells and B cells that recognize antigens previously encountered on exposure to pathogens or allergens. Beyond antigen specificity, the adaptive immune response is characterized by memory, whereby subsequent exposure to an antigen results in a much more rapid and robust immune response. For example, resident memory T cells patrol the skin and critically promote protective immunity in this manner.[1-3] However, in chronic inflammatory conditions such as psoriasis, this homeostatic process becomes pathologic.[4,5] Increasingly, it is becoming clear that, in addition to adaptive immune pathways, innate immune cells can also become dysfunctional and contribute to the pathogenesis of several inflammatory skin disorders.

The innate and adaptive immune systems can be subdivided into 3 major cell-mediated immune responses, termed type 1, type 2, and type 3 immunity. Type 1 immunity is mediated by adaptive T-helper type 1 (Th1) cells and cytotoxic T cells, as well as group 1 ILCs and natural killer cells. The primary function of the type 1 immune response, which is largely associated with interferon-$\gamma$ (IFN-$\gamma$) production, is to protect against intracellular pathogens and tumor cells. However, in cutaneous disorders, it plays a major role in the pathophysiology of ACD by mediating classic delayed-type hypersensitivity (DTH) reactions to haptens.[6]

The type 2 immune response is characterized by adaptive T-helper type 2 (Th2) cells, as well as innate basophils, eosinophils, group 2 ILCs (ILC2s), and mast cells. Collectively, these immune cells produce type 2 effector cytokines, including interleukin (IL)-4, IL-5, and IL-13. Briefly, IL-4 induces naive T-cell differentiation to Th2 cells, which in turn, along with IL-13, promotes class-switching of B cells to produce immunoglobulin (Ig) E. Generation of antigen-specific IgE is a key feature of allergic diseases such as AD and immediate type 1 hypersensitivity reactions such as urticaria. Further, IgE binds the high-affinity IgE receptor (Fc$\epsilon$RI) on both basophils and mast cells, serving as a bridge between adaptive (Th2 and B cells) and innate (basophils and mast cells) immunity. IL-5 is critical to eosinophil differentiation, activation, proliferation, and survival.[7,8] Although type 2 cytokine and IgE production normally promote expulsion of helminths and venoms, dysregulation of these homeostatic processes can also promote cutaneous inflammatory conditions such as AD and urticaria.[9-11]

Type 3 immunity is characterized by a predominance of adaptive T-helper type 17 (Th17) cells and gamma-delta T cells ($\gamma\delta$ T cells), as well as innate group 3 ILCs and neutrophils.[12,13] This immune axis is generally associated with the production of IL-17 and IL-22, which promote type 3 immune function by protecting against extracellular bacteria and fungi. Th17-cell overactivity is also well-established as a key driver of psoriasis pathophysiology, as shown by the remarkable efficacy of therapeutics targeting this pathway.[14-17] The growing understanding of the contribution of the cutaneous immune system to inflammatory skin disorders is continuing to show unprecedented value in informing the development of targeted therapeutics.[18,19] This article focuses on how recent innovations in the understanding of innate immunity have fundamentally changed paradigms of the pathogenesis of classic inflammatory skin disorders.

## TYPE 2 INFLAMMATION AND ATOPIC DERMATITIS

AD is a chronic and relapsing inflammatory skin disorder affecting up to 20% of children and 3% of adults worldwide.[20] In addition to hallmark oozing and crusted erythematous plaques, a central feature of AD is debilitating itch.[21,22] As with other atopic disorders with type 2 inflammatory pathologies, patients with AD are at increased risk for asthma, food allergy, and eosinophilic esophagitis, suggesting that systemic immune dysregulation is a core component of AD.[23–25] AD is at least partially defined by aberrant IgE production, allergen reactivity, and peripheral eosinophilia.[26,27] However, the precise contribution of IgE reactivity and eosinophils in AD remains unclear. Nevertheless, the role of type 2 cytokines in AD pathogenesis is now well established.

Classically, adaptive Th2 cells were long considered the primary drivers of AD pathogenesis through the production of IL-4 and IL-13.[28–30] However, in 2013, ILC2s were discovered in the skin of humans and mice, where they serve as a major source of type 2 cytokines and as mediators of murine AD-like disease.[31,32] Developmentally and functionally, ILC2s are similar to Th2 cells, but they lack antigen-specific receptors. Therefore, although they share similar transcriptional, phenotypic, and functional features with Th2 cell counterparts, they are classified as innate immune cells. In addition, basophils, which are not typically present in the skin, are recruited into lesional skin of both mice and humans with AD-associated inflammation, thereby promoting AD-like pathogenesis in mice. Taken together, these findings underscore that, beyond adaptive Th2 cells, various innate immune cell populations are also major sources of type 2 cytokines and likely contributors to AD pathogenesis.[33,34]

Although different clinical subtypes have been proposed, AD is now widely considered a predominantly type 2 cytokine–mediated disease.[35–37] Earlier studies postulated that AD was biphasic, with acute lesions showing type 2 activation signatures and chronic lesions skewing toward a type 1 response.[38,39] However, more recent transcriptional profiling studies suggest that the transition from acute to chronic inflammation in AD is characterized by quantitative rather than qualitative changes in cytokine profiles.[35] Notwithstanding possible immunologic heterogeneity, the efficacy and approval of dupilumab for moderate to severe AD in 2017 firmly established the receptor for IL-4 and IL-13 (IL-4Rα) as a major therapeutic target in AD pathogenesis (**Fig. 1**).[40] This pivotal scientific and clinical advance led to a major revolution in the drug development pipeline for AD. Beyond anti–IL-4Rα monoclonal antibody (mAb) blockade with dupilumab, 2 additional drugs are now in development for moderate to severe AD targeting IL-13. Both lebrikizumab and tralokinumab are anti–IL-13 mAbs that are currently in phase 3 clinical trials for moderate to severe AD (see **Fig. 1**).[41,42] Taken together, these major clinical advances have shown the importance of type 2 cytokines in AD pathogenesis.

For more than a decade, it was well known that overexpression of either IL-4 or IL-13 in mice led to AD-like disease and itch.[30,43] The efficacy of IL-4 and/or IL-13 blockade in patients with AD further confirmed the importance of these type 2 cytokines in the inflammatory pathogenesis of AD. However, the mechanisms driving itch in AD were elusive until recent years. IL-31 was the first cytokine shown to function as a pruritogen, or itch-inducing neurotransmitter, by directly stimulating sensory neurons to evoke itch.[44] Early murine studies showed that overexpression of IL-31 led to robust Th2-cell activation, resulting in severe dermatitis and pruritus.[45]

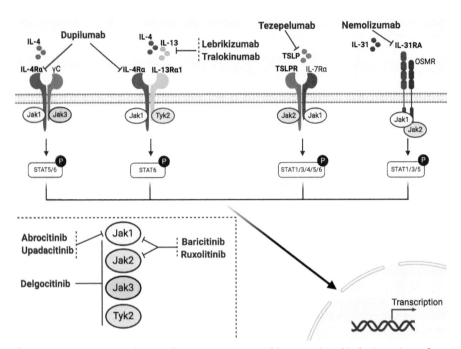

**Fig. 1.** Key immune signaling pathways in type 2 cytokine-associated itch. Overview of major signaling pathways associated with inflammatory itch in immune cells and sensory neurons. Therapeutic molecules currently in use, or under development, to modulate receptor signaling and downstream effectors (JAK inhibitors) are shown in red (antagonist). The image was created with BioRender. OSMR, oncostatin M receptor; STAT, signal transducer and activator of transcription; TSLP, thymic stromal lymphopoietin; TSLPR, thymic stromal lymphopoietin receptor.

Correspondingly, IL-31 expression is increased in lesional and nonlesional skin from patients with AD, and serum IL-31 levels correlate with disease severity across various AD subtypes.[46,47] More recently, phase 2 and 3 clinical trials with the anti–IL-31 receptor (IL-31RA) mAb, nemolizumab, have shown antipruritic efficacy in patients with AD (see **Fig. 1**).[48–50] Taken together, the biology and therapeutic impact of IL-31 blockade showed for the first time that a cytokine associated with AD directly engages the sensory nervous system to promote itch in a clinical meaningful way.

In 2017, Oetjen and colleagues[51] showed that IL-4Rα is expressed and functionally active on sensory neurons in mice and humans.[52,53] Findings from this study established that canonical type 2 cytokines, in addition to acting directly on the nervous system, can do so in a manner to promote neural hypersensitivity, or hyperknesis, to a variety of other pruritogens, including histamine.[51] This study showed how mAb-mediated blockade of IL-4Rα could broadly suppress neuronal hypersensitivity to relieve itch in patients with AD and other chronic pruritic disorders. Case reports and case series suggest that dupilumab may have the potential to effectively treat other itch disorders beyond AD, including uremic pruritus, malignancy-associated pruritus, prurigo nodularis, lichen planus, bullous pemphigoid, ACD, chronic spontaneous urticaria, and chronic pruritus of unknown origin.[54–57] Future studies will be required to determine to what extent these pruritogenic pathways overlap between AD and other chronic pruritic disorders.

Beyond the proven and evolving efficacy of blocking effector cytokines such as IL-4, IL-13, and IL-31 in AD pathogenesis, cytokines that function upstream of these pathways have also emerged as attractive therapeutic targets. Epithelial cell-derived cytokines such as IL-33 and thymic stromal lymphopoietin (TSLP) are secreted from stressed keratinocytes in the setting of AD-associated inflammation and act directly on a variety of cells, including Th2 cells and ILC2s, to promote type 2 inflammation.[29,32,58,59] Moreover, both IL-33 and TSLP act directly on sensory neurons and function as pruritogens too.[60,61] Consequently, mAbs targeting these cytokines (tezepelumab and etokimab) are currently under investigation in phase 2 clinical trials for treatment of AD (see **Fig. 1**).[60–62]

Although several different cytokines have been implicated in AD pathogenesis, many depend on downstream Janus kinase (JAK) signal transducer and activator of transcription (STAT) signaling cascades in lymphocytes and stromal cells for their activity. Thus, systemic JAK inhibition has emerged as a new therapeutic strategy for AD, with numerous agents now in phase 3 clinical trials, including abrocitinib (JAK1 inhibitor), baricitinib (JAK1/2 inhibitor), and upadacitinib (JAK1 inhibitor).[63–66] In sensory neurons, JAK1 represents an important downstream target because its deletion results in robust attenuation of itch.[51] Clinically, topical JAK inhibitors ruxolitinib (JAK1/2 inhibitor) and delgocitinib (pan-JAK inhibitor) have shown promising efficacy in AD and chronic hand dermatitis, respectively.[67–70] Altogether, these data point to a near future when JAK inhibitors will be US Food and Drug Administration–approved therapies for AD, and perhaps other pruritic disorders. By deciphering the neuroimmunologic basis of AD and its core symptoms, broader mechanisms of inflammation and itch are being revealed as targets for therapeutic intervention.

## ALLERGIC CONTACT DERMATITIS

ACD accounts for 20% of contact dermatoses and is considered a classic type IV hypersensitivity or DTH reaction, manifesting with pruritic eczematous lesions that occur hours to days after allergen exposure.[71] It progresses in 2 distinct phases: sensitization and elicitation. Sensitization is marked by epidermal penetration of an allergen or hapten, which is presented to allergen-specific naive T cells that then become activated and clonally expand to form memory T cells.[72,73] In the elicitation phase, allergen reexposure triggers circulating effector T cells to produce IFN-$\gamma$ and promote downstream inflammation.[74] In this manner, ACD is a paragon of adaptive antigen-specific Th1 disease, a paradigm originally proposed in the 1960s.

Despite the long-standing appreciation of adaptive DTH reactions in the pathogenesis of ACD, the mechanisms driving itch remained largely elusive until recently. More specifically, the pathways driving ACD-associated itch have yet to be directly correlated with the primary Th1 reaction. Recently, IL-33 was found to be markedly upregulated in the context of poison ivy (urushiol)–mediated ACD in mice, thus evoking itch by direct activation of its receptor on sensory neurons.[60] However, the mechanism by which IL-33 release is promoted in this context requires further elucidation. Similarly, another study, by Meixiong and colleagues,[75] identified upregulation of the neuropeptide pro-adrenomedullin N-terminal 20 peptide (PAMP) in the epidermis of inflamed ACD lesions from humans. In contrast with IL-33, however, PAMP mediates itch by mast cell activation, rather than direct stimulation of sensory neurons.[75]

The mast cell–nerve unit lies at the epicenter of itch biology. The mast cell has long been hailed as an integral driver of histamine-mediated or histaminergic itch, primarily through activation of IgE at its cell surface. However, in ACD, as in many other chronic itch disorders, antihistamines have proved largely ineffective as treatment modalities.[76] Further, IgE, although capable of binding peptide allergens, has no clear role in binding haptens to trigger ACD-associated inflammation. Thus, the role of mast cells in ACD remained largely unexplored until 2015, when the previously unrecognized murine Mas-related G protein–coupled receptor B2 (MRGPRB2) was found to be specifically expressed on mast cells.[77] This receptor is a member of the broader MRGPR family, which is strongly implicated in mediating itch, traditionally through neuronal expression of its family members (**Fig. 2**).[78,79] However, MRGPRB2 and its human ortholog, MRGPRX2, are among the only known MRGPRs expressed on non-neuronal tissues. They are both selectively expressed on mast cells and induce degranulation independently of IgE.[80,81] More specifically, MRGPRB2 and MRGPRX2 rapidly respond to a variety of endogenous peptide and exogenous peptidomimetic ligands, such as compound 48/80, which has been used to activate mast cells experimentally for more than 50 years.[77,82] Notably, it was the discovery of MRGPRB2 and MRGPRX2 that led to the identification of the receptor for 48/80. Strikingly, mast cell activation by compound 48/80 through MRGPRB2 results in histamine release comparable with IgE-mediated pathways, but other MRGPRB2 and MRGPRX2 ligands elicit different responses. MRGPRX2 is increasingly being identified as the target receptor for a growing number of compounds and medications associated with pseudoallergic drug reactions.[75,83,84] Thus, the discovery of MRGPRB2 and MRGPRX2

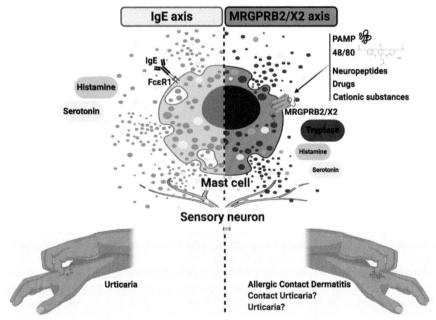

**Fig. 2.** IgE-mediated and MRGPRB2/X2-mediated mast cell activation at the neuroimmune interface. Mast cell activation by classic IgE-mediated pathways (*left*) results in the predominant release of histamine and serotonin, whereas mast cell activation by the MRGPRB2/X2 axis (*right*) can preferentially trigger the predominant release of other distinct mediators, such as tryptase, with markedly lower histamine and serotonin secretion. Emerging findings in cutaneous neuroimmunology are revealing novel pathways of MRGPRB2/X2-mediated itch in ACD triggered by neuropeptides (PAMP), peptidomimetic compounds (48/80, drugs) and haptens (cationic substances, drugs), which may also play a role in mediating nonhistaminergic itch in different forms of urticaria. The image was created with BioRender.

has opened up a major new area of inquiry into how mast cells may be uniquely activated to play novel roles in different disease states.

In patients with ACD, PAMP is upregulated in the epidermis in association with increased mast cell density in the dermis.[75] Correspondingly, PAMP is a ligand of mast cell–expressed MRGPRB2 and MRGPRX2. However, PAMP-mediated MRGPRB2–mast cell activation does not lead to robust histamine release as with classical IgE cross-linking at the cell surface.[85] Instead, mast cell degranulation along this axis leads to the preferential release of tryptase, a known pruritogen, suggesting a novel role for PAMP-MRGPRB2 signaling in mediating ACD-associated itch (see **Fig. 2**).[75] In support of this hypothesis, deletion of MRGPRB2 significantly reduced pruritis across 3 different murine models of ACD, further revealing a basis for mast cell–mediated nonhistaminergic itch in this disease context.[75] This concept was recently corroborated by Solinski and colleagues,[86] who showed that alternative modes of mast cell activation result in nonhistaminergic forms of itch as well. Taken together, these data support a model of ACD in which traditional DTH reactions drive the primary eczematous process, whereas itch is mediated secondarily by neuropeptides released from the epidermis to activate mast cell–mediated pruritis. Accordingly, future therapeutics designed to relieve ACD-associated itch may focus on the MRGPRX2–mast cell axis as a novel target.

## URTICARIA

Urticaria, or hives, is characterized by the onset of pruritic wheals that manifest as well-circumscribed areas of nonpitting edema with central pallor and raised borders involving the upper dermis. These fleeting lesions typically remit within 24 hours of onset and migrate if they recur. Although various causes have been identified, they are all categorized under 3 broad categories: allergic (food, medications, insects), nonallergic (mechanical or thermal stimuli), or idiopathic. Episodes lasting less than 6 weeks are classified as acute urticaria, whereas those lasting more than 6 weeks are categorized as chronic.[87] This distinction is significant because the underlying pathogenesis of each urticarial condition differs, as indicated by the disparate management of each.

Acute urticaria is the result of a classic type 1 hypersensitivity reaction. Briefly, a putative antigen binds to IgE on the surface of mast cells and basophils via FcεR1, cross-linking cell-bound IgE, and thereby driving mast cell and basophil activation and degranulation. The ensuing release of diverse preformed mediators, such as histamine, leads to enhanced vascular permeability and the delayed generation of cytokines that promote the physical and sensory manifestations of urticaria, such as itch.[88] In keeping with this pathophysiologic mechanism, acute urticaria is generally amenable to treatment with antihistamines.[89] However, a significant subset of acute urticaria is not responsive to antihistamines, suggesting other mechanisms of disease.

Chronic spontaneous urticaria (CSU) is a form of urticaria characterized by hallmark urticarial lesions irrespective of an inciting stimulus for a timespan greater than 6 weeks. In a subpopulation of patients, CSU is associated with circulating activating antibodies to IgE or its receptor FcεR1.[90] Patients with these and other chronic urticarias who show IgE reactivity can benefit from anti-IgE mAb treatment with omalizumab and ligelizumab, the latter currently in development, even when refractory to antihistamines.[91,92] However, many patients with CSU still do not respond to anti-IgE mAb therapy.[93] Given the lack of universal response to treatments along the IgE-histamine axis for a subset of patients with CSU, further investigation of other pathways, such as the MRGPRX2 axis, may represent an exciting new avenue for therapeutic intervention.

Contact urticaria is a form of acute urticaria characterized as a transient wheal-and-flare reaction that typically develops within minutes of exposure to an eliciting agent and usually resolves within 24 hours.[94] Although the immunologic variant of contact urticaria is derived from the IgE reactivity component, nonimmunologic contact urticaria is devoid of specific antibodies against the inciting agent. Antihistamines are therefore ineffective in treating nonimmunologic contact urticarial reactions, but a positive response to acetylsalicylic acid and nonsteroidal antiinflammatory drugs has been reported.[95,96] Interestingly, nonimmunologic contact urticarial reactions can also present with localized itching and redness without edema that generally remains localized to sites of contact. Given recent discoveries regarding mechanisms of MRGPRX2-mediated mast cell degranulation, it is possible that nonimmunologic contact urticaria may be a clinical manifestation of this form of IgE-independent mast cell activation. Further studies will be required to determine whether MRGPRX2 physiology underlies this mysterious form of contact urticaria.

## SUMMARY

Over the past 2 decades, the evolving therapeutic landscape of inflammatory cutaneous disorders has been largely driven by scientific advances in the understanding of skin immunology. In particular, seminal discoveries of the mechanisms underlying neuroimmune crosstalk have not only identified novel targets for medical intervention but also provided a rationale for the lack of efficacy associated with previous treatment modalities. The discovery of the MRGPRB2/X2–mast cell signaling axis, for example, has shed new light on the shortcomings of IgE and histamine blockade in treating pruritic disorders such as ACD, while simultaneously opening new lines of inquiry into the potential contribution of MRGPRB2/X2 biology in the context of CSU and contact urticaria. Just as JAK inhibitors are currently on the cusp of redefining the management of chronic inflammatory skin orders, so too may MRGPRB2/X2 immunomodulatory agents soon emerge at the cutting edge of dermatology and clinical allergy and immunology in the years to come.

## CLINICS CARE POINTS

- Type 2 cytokine blockade has shown favorable safety and unique efficacy in AD.
- Type 2 cytokine blockade and JAK inhibition may have broader applications well beyond AD toward other chronic itch disorders.
- Targeting of T cell–independent and IgE-independent mechanisms on mast cells (eg, MRGPRX2) likely represents new therapeutic strategies for itch associated with ACD and urticaria.

## DISCLOSURE

B.S. Kim has served as a consultant for AbbVie, ABRAX Japan, Almirall, AstraZeneca, Cara Therapeutics, Daewoong Pharmaceutical, Incyte, LEO Pharma, Lilly, Maruho, Menlo Therapeutics, OM Pharma, Pfizer, and Third Rock Ventures. He has also participated on the advisory board for Almirall, Boehringer Ingelheim, Cara Therapeutics, Kiniksa Pharmaceuticals, Menlo Therapeutics, Regeneron Pharmaceuticals, Sanofi Genzyme, and Trevi Therapeutics. He is stockholder of Locus Biosciences. All other authors declare that they have no relevant conflicts of interest.

## REFERENCES

1. Jiang X, Clark RA, Liu L, et al. Skin infection generates non-migratory memory CD8+ T(RM) cells providing global skin immunity. Nature 2012;483:227–31.
2. Mueller SN, Mackay LK. Tissue-resident memory T cells: local specialists in immune defence. Nat Rev Immunol 2016;16:79–89.
3. Ho AW, Kupper TS. T cells and the skin: from protective immunity to inflammatory skin disorders. Nat Rev Immunol 2019;19:490–502.
4. Matos TR, O'Malley JT, Lowry EL, et al. Clinically resolved psoriatic lesions contain psoriasis-specific IL-17-producing αβ T cell clones. J Clin Invest 2017; 127:4031–41.
5. Pan Y, Tian T, Park CO, et al. Survival of tissue-resident memory T cells requires exogenous lipid uptake and metabolism. Nature 2017;543:252–6.
6. Annunziato F, Romagnani C, Romagnani S. The 3 major types of innate and adaptive cell-mediated effector immunity. J Allergy Clin Immunol 2015;135:626–35.
7. Gandhi NA, Bennett BL, Graham NM, et al. Targeting key proximal drivers of type 2 inflammation in disease. Nat Rev Drug Discov 2016;15:35–50.
8. Romagnani S. Lymphokine production by human T cells in disease states. Annu Rev Immunol 1994;12:227–57.
9. Allen JE, Sutherland TE. Host protective roles of type 2 immunity: parasite killing and tissue repair, flip sides of the same coin. Semin Immunol 2014;26:329–40.
10. Palm NW, Rosenstein RK, Yu S, et al. Bee venom phospholipase A2 induces a primary type 2 response that is dependent on the receptor ST2 and confers protective immunity. Immunity 2013;39:976–85.
11. Galli SJ, Starkl P, Marichal T, et al. Mast cells and IgE in defense against venoms: Possible "good side" of allergy? Allergol Int 2016;65:3–15.
12. Harrington LE, Hatton RD, Mangan PR, et al. Interleukin 17-producing CD4+ effector T cells develop via a lineage distinct from the T helper type 1 and 2 lineages. Nat Immunol 2005;6:1123–32.
13. Rutz S, Eidenschenk C, Ouyang W. IL-22, not simply a Th17 cytokine. Immunol Rev 2013;252:116–32.
14. Marinoni B, Ceribelli A, Massarotti MS, et al. The Th17 axis in psoriatic disease: pathogenetic and therapeutic implications. Auto Immun Highlights 2014;5:9–19.
15. Eberle FC, Brück J, Holstein J, et al. Recent advances in understanding psoriasis. F1000Research 2016;5. F1000 Faculty Rev-770.
16. Dyring-Andersen B, Honoré TV, Madelung A, et al. Interleukin (IL)-17A and IL-22-producing neutrophils in psoriatic skin. Br J Dermatol 2017;177:e321–2.
17. Menter A, Strober BE, Kaplan DH, et al. Joint AAD-NPF guidelines of care for the management and treatment of psoriasis with biologics. J Am Acad Dermatol 2019;80:1029–72.
18. Erickson S, Nahmias Z, Rosman IS, et al. Immunomodulating agents as antipruritics. Dermatol Clin 2018;36:325–34.
19. Billi AC, Gudjonsson JE, Voorhees JJ. Psoriasis: past, present, and future. J Invest Dermatol 2019;139:e133–42.
20. Asher MI, Montefort S, Björkstén B, et al. Worldwide time trends in the prevalence of symptoms of asthma, allergic rhinoconjunctivitis, and eczema in childhood: ISAAC Phases One and Three repeat multicountry cross-sectional surveys. Lancet 2006;368:733–43.
21. Kini SP, DeLong LK, Veledar E, et al. The impact of pruritus on quality of life: the skin equivalent of pain. Arch Dermatol 2011;147:1153–6.

22. Yosipovitch G, Bernhard JD. Clinical practice. Chronic pruritus. N Engl J Med 2013;368:1625–34.
23. Silverberg JI. Comorbidities and the impact of atopic dermatitis. Ann Allergy Asthma Immunol 2019;123:144–51.
24. Silverberg JI, Gelfand JM, Margolis DJ, et al. Patient burden and quality of life in atopic dermatitis in US adults: A population-based cross-sectional study. Ann Allergy Asthma Immunol 2018;121:340–7.
25. Hill DA, Spergel JM. The immunologic mechanisms of eosinophilic esophagitis. Curr Allergy Asthma Rep 2016;16:9.
26. Liu FT, Goodarzi H, Chen HY. IgE, mast cells, and eosinophils in atopic dermatitis. Clin Rev Allergy Immunol 2011;41:298–310.
27. Jenerowicz D, Czarnecka-Operacz M, Silny W. Peripheral blood eosinophilia in atopic dermatitis. Acta Dermatovenerol Alp Pannonica Adriat 2007;16:47–52.
28. Hamid Q, Boguniewicz M, Leung DY. Differential in situ cytokine gene expression in acute versus chronic atopic dermatitis. J Clin Invest 1994;94:870–6.
29. Soumelis V, Reche PA, Kanzler H, et al. Human epithelial cells trigger dendritic cell mediated allergic inflammation by producing TSLP. Nat Immunol 2002;3:673–80.
30. Chan LS, Robinson N, Xu L. Expression of interleukin-4 in the epidermis of transgenic mice results in a pruritic inflammatory skin disease: an experimental animal model to study atopic dermatitis. J Invest Dermatol 2001;117:977–83.
31. Roediger B, Kyle R, Yip KH, et al. Cutaneous immunosurveillance and regulation of inflammation by group 2 innate lymphoid cells. Nat Immunol 2013;14:564–73.
32. Kim BS, Siracusa MC, Saenz SA, et al. TSLP elicits IL-33-independent innate lymphoid cell responses to promote skin inflammation. Sci Transl Med 2013;5:170ra16.
33. Poposki JA, Klingler AI, Tan BK, et al. Group 2 innate lymphoid cells are elevated and activated in chronic rhinosinusitis with nasal polyps. Immun Inflamm Dis 2017;5:233–43.
34. Martinez-Gonzalez I, Steer CA, Takei F. Lung ILC2s link innate and adaptive responses in allergic inflammation. Trends Immunol 2015;36:189–95.
35. Tsoi LC, Rodriguez E, Stölzl D, et al. Progression of acute-to-chronic atopic dermatitis is associated with quantitative rather than qualitative changes in cytokine responses. J Allergy Clin Immunol 2020;145:1406–15.
36. Bieber T, D'Erme AM, Akdis CA, et al. Clinical phenotypes and endophenotypes of atopic dermatitis: Where are we, and where should we go? J Allergy Clin Immunol 2017;139:S58–64.
37. Brunner PM, Guttman-Yassky E, Leung DY. The immunology of atopic dermatitis and its reversibility with broad-spectrum and targeted therapies. J Allergy Clin Immunol 2017;139:S65–76.
38. Thepen T, Langeveld-Wildschut EG, Bihari IC, et al. Biphasic response against aeroallergen in atopic dermatitis showing a switch from an initial TH2 response to a TH1 response in situ: an immunocytochemical study. J Allergy Clin Immunol 1996;97:828–37.
39. Grewe M, Gyufko K, Schöpf E, et al. Lesional expression of interferon-gamma in atopic eczema. Lancet 1994;343:25–6.
40. Simpson EL, Bieber T, Guttman-Yassky E, et al. Two Phase 3 Trials of dupilumab versus placebo in atopic dermatitis. N Engl J Med 2016;375:2335–48.
41. Guttman-Yassky E, Blauvelt A, Eichenfield LF, et al. Efficacy and safety of lebrikizumab, a high-affinity interleukin 13 inhibitor, in adults with moderate to severe

atopic dermatitis: a phase 2b randomized clinical trial. JAMA Dermatol 2020;156: 411–20.

42. Uppal SK, Kearns DG, Chat VS, et al. Review and analysis of biologic therapies currently in phase II and phase III clinical trials for atopic dermatitis. J Dermatol Treat 2020;1–11. https://doi.org/10.1080/09546634.2020.1775775.

43. Zheng T, Oh MH, Oh SY, et al. Transgenic expression of interleukin-13 in the skin induces a pruritic dermatitis and skin remodeling. J Invest Dermatol 2009;129: 742–51.

44. Cevikbas F, Wang X, Akiyama T, et al. A sensory neuron-expressed IL-31 receptor mediates T helper cell-dependent itch: Involvement of TRPV1 and TRPA1. J Allergy Clin Immunol 2014;133:448–60.

45. Dillon SR, Sprecher C, Hammond A, et al. Interleukin 31, a cytokine produced by activated T cells, induces dermatitis in mice. Nat Immunol 2004;5:752–60.

46. Sonkoly E, Muller A, Lauerma AI, et al. IL-31: a new link between T cells and pruritus in atopic skin inflammation. J Allergy Clin Immunol 2006;117:411–7.

47. Raap U, Wichmann K, Bruder M, et al. Correlation of IL-31 serum levels with severity of atopic dermatitis. J Allergy Clin Immunol 2008;122:421–3.

48. Nemoto O, Furue M, Nakagawa H, et al. The first trial of CIM331, a humanized antihuman interleukin-31 receptor A antibody, in healthy volunteers and patients with atopic dermatitis to evaluate safety, tolerability and pharmacokinetics of a single dose in a randomized, double-blind, placebo-controlled study. Br J Dermatol 2016;174:296–304.

49. Ruzicka T, Mihara R. Anti-Interleukin-31 Receptor A Antibody for Atopic Dermatitis. N Engl J Med 2017;376:2093.

50. Kabashima K, Matsumura T, Komazaki H, et al. Trial of nemolizumab and topical agents for atopic dermatitis with pruritus. N Engl J Med 2020;383:141–50.

51. Oetjen LK, Mack MR, Feng J, et al. Sensory neurons co-opt classical immune signaling pathways to mediate chronic itch. Cell 2017;171:217–28.e13.

52. Usoskin D, Furlan A, Islam S, et al. Unbiased classification of sensory neuron types by large-scale single-cell RNA sequencing. Nat Neurosci 2015;18:145–53.

53. Mueller TD, Zhang JL, Sebald W, et al. Structure, binding, and antagonists in the IL-4/IL-13 receptor system. Biochim Biophys Acta 2002;1592:237–50.

54. Holm JG, Agner T, Sand C, et al. Dupilumab for prurigo nodularis: Case series and review of the literature. Dermatol Ther 2020;33:e13222.

55. Zhai LL, Savage KT, Qiu CC, et al. Chronic pruritus responding to dupilumab-a case series. Medicines (Basel) 2019;6:72.

56. Hendricks AJ, Yosipovitch G, Shi VY. Dupilumab use in dermatologic conditions beyond atopic dermatitis - a systematic review. J Dermatol Treat 2019;32(1): 19–28.

57. Seidman JS, Eichenfield DZ, Orme CM. Dupilumab for bullous pemphigoid with intractable pruritus. Dermatol Online J 2019;25. 13030/qt25q9w6r9.

58. Imai Y, Yasuda K, Sakaguchi Y, et al. Skin-specific expression of IL-33 activates group 2 innate lymphoid cells and elicits atopic dermatitis-like inflammation in mice. Proc Natl Acad Sci U S A 2013;110:13921–6.

59. Leyva-Castillo JM, Hener P, Jiang H, et al. TSLP produced by keratinocytes promotes allergen sensitization through skin and thereby triggers atopic march in mice. J Invest Dermatol 2013;133:154–63.

60. Liu B, Tai Y, Achanta S, et al. IL-33/ST2 signaling excites sensory neurons and mediates itch response in a mouse model of poison ivy contact allergy. Proc Natl Acad Sci U S A 2016;113:E7572.e9.

61. Wilson SR, Thé L, Batia LM, et al. The epithelial cell-derived atopic dermatitis cytokine TSLP activates neurons to induce itch. Cell 2013;155:285–95.
62. Chen YL, Gutowska-Owsiak D, Hardman CS, et al. Proof-of-concept clinical trial of etokimab shows a key role for IL-33 in atopic dermatitis pathogenesis. Sci Transl Med 2019;11. eaax2945.
63. Gooderham MJ, Forman SB, Bissonnette R, et al. Efficacy and safety of oral janus kinase 1 inhibitor abrocitinib for patients with atopic dermatitis: a phase 2 randomized clinical trial. JAMA Dermatol 2019;155:1371–9.
64. Simpson EL, Lacour JP, Spelman L, et al. Baricitinib in patients with moderate-to-severe atopic dermatitis and inadequate response to topical corticosteroids: results from two randomized monotherapy phase III trials. Br J Dermatol 2020;183: 242–55.
65. Guttman-Yassky E, Silverberg JI, Nemoto O, et al. Baricitinib in adult patients with moderate-to-severe atopic dermatitis: A phase 2 parallel, double-blinded, randomized placebo-controlled multiple-dose study. J Am Acad Dermatol 2019; 80:913–21.e9.
66. Guttman-Yassky E, Thaçi D, Pangan AL, et al. Upadacitinib in adults with moderate to severe atopic dermatitis: 16-week results from a randomized, placebo-controlled trial. J Allergy Clin Immunol 2020;145:877–84.
67. Kim BS, Sun K, Papp K, et al. Effects of ruxolitinib cream on pruritus and quality of life in atopic dermatitis: Results from a phase 2, randomized, dose-ranging, vehicle- and active-controlled study. J Am Acad Dermatol 2020;82:1305–13.
68. Kim BS, Howell MD, Sun K, et al. Treatment of atopic dermatitis with ruxolitinib cream (JAK1/JAK2 inhibitor) or triamcinolone cream. J Allergy Clin Immunol 2020;145:572–82.
69. Worm M, Bauer A, Elsner P, et al. Efficacy and safety of topical delgocitinib in patients with chronic hand eczema: data from a randomized, double-blind, vehicle-controlled phase IIa study. Br J Dermatol 2020;182:1103–10.
70. Nakagawa H, Nemoto O, Igarashi A, et al. Phase 2 clinical study of delgocitinib ointment in pediatric patients with atopic dermatitis. J Allergy Clin Immunol 2019; 144:1575–83.
71. Kostner L, Anzengruber F, Guillod C, et al. Allergic Contact Dermatitis. Immunol Allergy Clin North Am 2017;37:141–52.
72. Kaplan DH, Jenison MC, Saeland S, et al. Epidermal langerhans cell-deficient mice develop enhanced contact hypersensitivity. Immunity 2005;23:611–20.
73. Seneschal J, Clark RA, Gehad A, et al. Human epidermal Langerhans cells maintain immune homeostasis in skin by activating skin resident regulatory T cells. Immunity 2012;36:873–84.
74. Saint-Mezard P, Krasteva M, Chavagnac C, et al. Afferent and efferent phases of allergic contact dermatitis (ACD) can be induced after a single skin contact with haptens: evidence using a mouse model of primary ACD. J Invest Dermatol 2003; 120:641–7.
75. Meixiong J, Anderson M, Limjunyawong N, et al. Activation of mast-cell-expressed mas-related g-protein-coupled receptors drives non-histaminergic itch. Immunity 2019;50:1163–71.e5.
76. Kamo A, Negi O, Tengara S, et al. Histamine H(4) receptor antagonists ineffective against itch and skin inflammation in atopic dermatitis mouse model. J Invest Dermatol 2014;134:546–8.
77. McNeil BD, Pundir P, Meeker S, et al. Identification of a mast-cell-specific receptor crucial for pseudo-allergic drug reactions. Nature 2015;519:237–41.

78. Dong X, Han S, Zylka MJ, et al. A diverse family of GPCRs expressed in specific subsets of nociceptive sensory neurons. Cell 2001;106:619–32.
79. Liu Q, Tang Z, Surdenikova L, et al. Sensory neuron-specific GPCR Mrgprs are itch receptors mediating chloroquine-induced pruritus. Cell 2009;139:1353–65.
80. Kashem SW, Subramanian H, Collington SJ, et al. G protein coupled receptor specificity for C3a and compound 48/80-induced degranulation in human mast cells: roles of Mas-related genes MrgX1 and MrgX2. Eur J Pharmacol 2011; 668:299–304.
81. Tatemoto K, Nozaki Y, Tsuda R, et al. Immunoglobulin E-independent activation of mast cell is mediated by Mrg receptors. Biochem Biophys Res Commun 2006; 349:1322–8.
82. Subramanian H, Gupta K, Guo Q, et al. Mas-related gene X2 (MrgX2) is a novel G protein-coupled receptor for the antimicrobial peptide LL-37 in human mast cells: resistance to receptor phosphorylation, desensitization, and internalization. J Biol Chem 2011;286:44739–49.
83. Navinés-Ferrer A, Serrano-Candelas E, Lafuente A, et al. MRGPRX2-mediated mast cell response to drugs used in perioperative procedures and anaesthesia. Sci Rep 2018;8:11628.
84. Subramanian H, Gupta K, Ali H. Roles of Mas-related G protein-coupled receptor X2 on mast cell-mediated host defense, pseudoallergic drug reactions, and chronic inflammatory diseases. J Allergy Clin Immunol 2016;138:700–10.
85. Kamohara M, Matsuo A, Takasaki J, et al. Identification of MrgX2 as a human G-protein-coupled receptor for proadrenomedullin N-terminal peptides. Biochem Biophys Res Commun 2005;330:1146–52.
86. Solinski HJ, Kriegbaum MC, Tseng PY, et al. Nppb neurons are sensors of mast cell-induced itch. Cell Rep 2019;26:3561–73.e4.
87. Zuberbier T, Aberer W, Asero R, et al. The EAACI/GA$^2$LEN/EDF/WAO guideline for the definition, classification, diagnosis and management of urticaria. Allergy 2018;73:1393–414.
88. Dvorak AM. New aspects of mast cell biology. Int Arch Allergy Immunol 1997; 114:1–9.
89. Zuberbier T, Iffländer J, Semmler C, et al. Acute urticaria: clinical aspects and therapeutic responsiveness. Acta Derm Venereol 1996;76:295–7.
90. Vasagar K, Vonakis BM, Gober LM, et al. Evidence of in vivo basophil activation in chronic idiopathic urticaria. Clin Exp Allergy 2006;36:770–6.
91. Maurer M, Rosén K, Hsieh HJ, et al. Omalizumab for the treatment of chronic idiopathic or spontaneous urticaria. N Engl J Med 2013;368:924–35.
92. Maurer M, Giménez-Arnau AM, Sussman G, et al. Ligelizumab for Chronic Spontaneous Urticaria. N Engl J Med 2019;381:1321–32.
93. Khan S, Sholtysek S. Omalizumab re-treatment rates in chronic spontaneous urticaria. Eur Ann Allergy Clin Immunol 2020;52:187–9.
94. Vethachalam S, Persaud Y. Contact urticaria. StatPearls. Treasure Island (FL): StatPearls Publishing Copyright © 2020, StatPearls Publishing LLC.; 2020.
95. Venarske D, deShazo RD. Molecular mechanisms of allergic disease. South Med J 2003;96:1049–54.
96. Novembre E, Cianferoni A, Mori F, et al. Urticaria and urticaria related skin condition/disease in children. Eur Ann Allergy Clin Immunol 2008;40:5–13.

# Advances in the Translational Science of Dermatitis

Sara Bilimoria, MS, Kyle Tegtmeyer, BS, Peter Lio, MD*

## KEYWORDS

• Atopic dermatitis • Translational medicine • Therapeutics • Pathophysiology

## KEY POINTS

- There is much than remains unknown about the translational science of dermatitis. There is significant overlap of genetic and environmental barrier disruption. Barrier disruption influences sensitization to protein allergens including commensal organisms (in atopic dermatitis) versus nonprotein allergens (in what is referred to as allergic contact dermatitis).
- The identification of key cytokines such as interleukin (IL)-4 and IL-13, along with the JAK-STAT signaling pathway, has provided potential therapeutic targets.
- The first targeted biologic agents and selective oral agents are finally available or will be imminently, and the pipeline is robust.

## INTRODUCTION

The National Institutes of Health (NIH) National Center for Advancing Translational Sciences defines translation as "the process of turning observations in the laboratory, clinic, and community into interventions that improve the health of individuals and the public."[1] Dermatitis has seemingly resisted translational breakthroughs, while other inflammatory diseases such as psoriasis, rheumatoid arthritis, and inflammatory bowel disease have seen extraordinary advances in targeted therapeutics, with commensurate impacts on disease outcomes and quality of life.[2,3] (**Fig. 1**).

Despite a backdrop of tremendous and rapidly increasing basic scientific knowledge about dermatitis, in 2013 Professor Hywel Williams pointed out 7 areas of notable ignorance, including 2 areas questioning the fundamental nosology and ontology of the disease: "Is atopic dermatitis (AD) more than one disease?" and "What causes AD to flare?"[4] It is perhaps not surprising then, that the integral cycle of development for translational medicine was somewhat stuck at the very beginning, unable to progress until pathophysiology could be elucidated and targets selected

Northwestern University Feinberg School of Medicine, 363 West Erie Street, Suite 350, Chicago, IL 60616, USA
* Corresponding author.
*E-mail address:* peterlio@gmail.com

Immunol Allergy Clin N Am 41 (2021) 361–373
https://doi.org/10.1016/j.iac.2021.04.001
0889-8561/21/© 2021 Elsevier Inc. All rights reserved.                immunology.theclinics.com

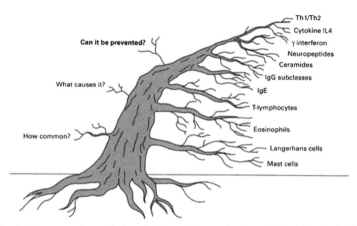

**Fig. 1.** The listing tree of translational science in atopic dermatitis. AD, atopic dermatitis; IgE, immunoglobulin E; Th2, T helper 2. (*From* Williams HC. *Atopic Dermatitis: The Epidemiology, Causes and Prevention of Atopic Eczema.* Cambridge University Press; 2000; with permission.)

(**Fig. 2**). Much work is currently underway investigating treatments targeting the many immunologic facets of AD, and addressing concerns such as skin barrier integrity and the skin microbiome, with an albeit incomplete understanding of the underlying pathophysiology of AD.

## BARRIER DYSFUNCTION

Barrier dysfunction is a central component of dermatitis pathobiology and a potential target for clinical management. In both the lesional and nonlesional skin areas of patients with AD, a compromised skin barrier allows for irritant, allergen, and pathogen penetration, increasing the risk of infection and allergic sensitization.[5] The skin barrier is often conceived as simply a physical barrier, but has critical functional activities also, including microbiome, chemical, and immunologic

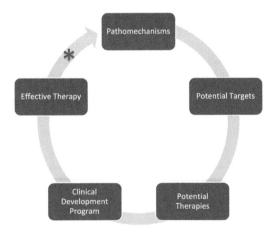

**Fig. 2.** The virtuous cycle moving from pathomechanisms to effective therapies. The star denotes feedback about the pathogenesis of a disease by understanding why a therapy is effective, sometimes referred to as *diagnosis ex juvantibus.*

homeostatis.[6] A skin barrier discussion is incomplete without considering filaggrin, a key protein found in the stratum corneum responsible for the health of individual corneocytes and their structural integrity. Filaggrin, encoded by the *FLG* gene, is metabolized into amino acids, which are part of the natural moisturizing factors that contribute to epidermal hydration and acidity.[7] It is widely accepted that filaggrin dysfunction and AD are closely related, but it is unclear which comes first: does filaggrin dysfunction predispose to AD, or does the inflammatory environment of AD induce the barrier dysfunction cascade? It is now understood that it does not matter which comes first, because the barrier is universally disrupted in AD.[8] Accordingly, to improve barrier dysfunction, the specific aspect or aspects can theoretically be targeted.

Moisturizers are a cornerstone of AD therapy, underpinning various topical and systemic therapies for optimal control. Moisturizers primarily comprise 3 components: humectants, occlusives, and emollients. Humectants attract water from the epidermis and dermis to the stratum corneum, occlusives form a physical barrier over the stratum corneum to prevent transepidermal water loss (TEWL), and emollients help fill gaps between corneocytes to smooth the skin. Although it is well- and long-suggested that moisturizers are effective for existing AD, there are few comparative studies to help guide selection of an optimal moisturizer, let alone a precision choice to address a targeted defect in a given patient.[9–11]

Randomized trials have been conducted to determine the protective utility of applying moisturizers to newborns' skin to prevent AD development in infancy and childhood. One study found daily emollient use reduced the incidence of AD with only 6 months of use,[12] but follow-up studies have not replicated this finding.[13,14] Similarly, use of slightly acidic ceramide-rich emollients on newborns reduced risk of both AD development and food sensitization, spurred by the concept of transcutaneous sensitization as a primary mechanism of pathogenesis.[15] Presently, it appears that targeting AD through skin barrier maintenance, repair, and protection with moisturizers may be important for preventing allergic sensitization and atopy; research indicates this may be optimal in infancy and childhood.[16,17]

## SKIN MICROBIOME

The skin surface prevents dangerous colonization and infection by pathogens by maintaining a delicately balanced microbiome. Current research indicates that increased concentrations of *Staphylococcus aureus* can exacerbate disease through heightened inflammation and allergic sensitization, both of which are mediated by various virulence factors and direct effects on keratinocytes.[18]

Bacterial adherence appears to be increased in AD skin, and adhesins represent a virulence factor that *S aureus* uses to enhance adherence.[19] *S aureus* also releases various cell-damaging and immune-activating exotoxins that weaken the skin barrier integrity and enable invasion and dissemination to host skin. This effect is particularly prominent in patients with an already compromised skin barrier such as AD patients. Some of these toxins act as superantigens, binding and activating multiple T cells at once, regardless of T cell receptor specificity. This aberrant T cell activation can cause uncontrolled release of inflammatory mediators and contribute to the morbidity of AD.[20,21]

Allergic contact dermatitis (ACD) is a cutaneous cell-mediated hypersensitivity reaction instigated by environmental allergens. In ACD, allergens bind carrier proteins and form complexes, which elicit an inflammatory response similar to that found in AD.[22] Treatment benefits for AD may be augmented by diagnosing and avoiding contact allergens.[23]

Advances in metagenomic sequencing for whole-microbiome analysis and preclinical studies of transplanted lesional flora in mice have significantly advanced the understanding of the skin microbiome and its impact on dermatitis. This improved understanding has allowed for advances in therapeutics that reverse dysbiosis through introduction of commensal species.

Therapeutic targeting of aberrant *S aureus* colonization is the basis of several clinical trials involving topical corticosteroids, antibiotics, and other antimicrobial approaches. In a randomized placebo-controlled trial of pediatric AD patients, treatment with a 2-week course of cephalexin with or without intranasal mupirocin and a sodium hypochlorite bath compared with intranasal petroleum ointment and a plain water bath led to significant reductions in the Eczema Area and Severity Index score (EASI) at 1 and 3 months.[24] Although the role of the dilute bleach bath has now been elucidated to likely be anti-inflammatory,[25] antipruritic, and possibly improving barrier function,[26] it seems settled that it is not actually antimicrobial in this context.[27–29]

Studies into the role of commensal organisms in normal skin homeostasis and dysbiosis have opened the door to a new modality of targeting the microbiome for therapy. It has been shown that introduction of commensal *Staphylococcus epidermidis* species to neonatal skin during a critical period for colonization induces a regulatory T cell response that promotes later immune recognition and dampening of aberrant inflammatory responses to specific species.[30] Recently, results of a small open-label trial of *Roseomonas mucosa* as a commensal bacteria-based treatment of AD showed improvement in a pediatric cohort for SCORAD, EASI, and clinical endpoints at 4 months following a dose-escalation regimen and a fixed dose of $10^5$ CFU.[31] Although early research has shown promise, future study is needed for the development of skin microbiome therapeutics and commensal bacteria delivery strategies that can be more broadly applied to dermatitis patients in a clinical setting.

## BIOLOGICS/IMMUNE TARGETS
### Inhibition of Th2 Responses

Lesional tissue from acute AD is characterized by a polarization toward Th2-predominant inflammatory profiles, with increased expression of the cytokines IL-4, IL-5, IL-13, and IL-31.[32] The overabundance of cytokines can wreak havoc on the immune system by triggering an inflammatory cascade along with the downregulation of terminal differentiation genes and tight junction products, all of which are essential for skin barrier integrity. AD patients have compromised skin barriers likely due in part to the surge of cytokines suppressing these protective mechanisms. Antibody-mediated inhibition of these interleukins may hinder the inflammatory Th2 pathway enough to inhibit pathogenesis of AD.[33,34] Several monoclonal antibodies target the Th2 pathway and are being studied or are US Food and Drug Administration (FDA)-approved for the treatment of AD.

### Interleukin-5

IL-5 plays a role in the activation, growth, differentiation, and recruitment of eosinophils to lesional tissue in AD. Its expression is highest in chronic lesions, with T cells comprising the largest population of IL-5 expressing cells in acute and chronic lesions.[32,35] Mice with knockout of IL-5 have pronounced decreases in cutaneous eosinophilia and epidermal thickening in response to allergen exposure.[36]

Mepolizumab is a humanized IgG monoclonal antibody with binding affinity for IL-5. Mepolizumab has been found to reduce baseline blood eosinophil counts, a mechanism that has potential in reducing inflammation in AD.[37] When given to patients with

AD, mepolizumab showed notable improvements in erythema, infiltration, and papulation, but no notable reduction in dermatitis or pruritus.[38] Similarly, a multicenter trial treating adult patients with moderate-to-severe AD with mepolizumab did not show significant clinical improvement, but did demonstrate a reduction in blood eosinophil levels. This suggests that serum eosinophils may have negligible impact on tissue-bound eosinophils relevant in the pathology of AD, and that anti IL-5 therapy may be less effective in treating AD than initially thought.[39,40]

### Interleukin-31
IL-31 is a known contributing factor to pruritus in AD. This has been demonstrated by the AD-like irritation caused by increased IL-31 expression engineered in mice.[41] In AD patients, there appears to be a strong correlation between circulating IL-31 and phenotypic severity of skin disease.[42,43] Furthermore, patients with AD are thought to be more sensitive to serum IL-31, as their keratinocytes have increased expression of IL-31 receptors.[44] IL-31 is also noted to interfere with keratinocyte proliferation and suppress filaggrin expression.[45] Together, these findings are evidence of IL-31's significant role in AD pathophysiology.

Given the significant role of IL-31 in the pathophysiology of AD as the previously mentioned studies suggest, targeting IL-31 with a monoclonal antibody presents a particularly attractive therapeutic option. Nemolizumab, a monoclonal antibody against the IL-31 receptor, has shown clinical efficacy in treating AD. A phase 2b randomized-controlled trial found that subcutaneous nemolizumab dosed every 4 weeks for 24 weeks significantly improved EASI scores ($P=.016$) and NRS-itch scores ($P\leq.01$). Nemolizumab was successful in reducing inflammation and providing rapid and sustained pruritus relief. The success of nemolizumab in controlling IL-31 activity suggests it may be a potential therapy for ACD also, as there appear to be elevated levels of IL-31 in ACD patients.[46] Nemolizumab has been granted breakthrough therapy designation from the FDA, allowing expedited research and development in the therapy.[47,48]

### Interleukin-33
IL-33 contributes to eczematous inflammation by acting as an alarmin, mediating the activation of the adaptive immune system by promoting Th2 and Th1 responses. IL-33 has also been shown to have barrier-weakening properties. One study observed the direct action of IL-33 on downregulation of *FLG* gene expression. Further, there was stronger *FLG* suppression in cells derived from patients with AD than in cells derived from healthy donors, suggesting AD skin is more prone to filaggrin dysregulation by IL-33 than healthy skin.[49]

Studies targeting IL-33 have not yet shown significant promise in the treatment of AD. One such monoclonal antibody targeting IL-33, etokimab, failed to achieve its primary endpoint of significant improvement in EASI score across all treatment arms in the ATLAS trial, per reports from its manufacturer.[50] Because of disappointing initial results and more promising therapeutic options in development, future study and development of IL-33 inhibition for AD therapy do not appear likely at this time.

### Interleukin-4 and interleukin-13
IL-4 and IL-13 are cytokines produced by Th2 lymphocytes that are central to the pathogenesis of allergic diseases and asthma. Both cytokines have increased expression in AD patients and are proinflammatory.[51,52] IL-4 and IL-13 facilitate hypersensitivity reactions by promoting IgE production, leading to inflammation in skin and blood. Therefore, targeting IL-4 and IL-13 has been attempted for the treatment of AD.

Dupilumab is a monoclonal antibody that targets the common, shared portion of the IL-4 and IL-13 receptors–the IL-4 receptor alpha subunit–and has been studied and approved for the treatment of AD.[53]

In a phase 3 study in which dupilumab monotherapy was compared with a placebo intervention, dupilumab was significantly superior in achieving a clear or almost clear global assessment at 16 weeks. In addition, the dupilumab group reported improvements in pruritus and symptoms of anxiety and depression, factors that significantly compromise quality of life in AD patients.[54] Children and adolescents are some of the most heavily burdened AD patients with similar challenges to quality of life as adults in addition to the mental and social repercussions of visible disease. A phase 3 study assessing dupilumab in adolescents ($\geq$12 years) with moderate-to-severe AD supported use of the biologic agent in this population with no new safety concerns.[55] In 2019, the FDA approved dose-adjusted dupilumab therapy for patients aged 12 to 17 years with moderate-to-severe uncontrolled AD. Soon after, another clinical trial resulted in FDA approval of dupilumab for children aged 6 to 11 years with moderate-to-severe AD.[56]

The utility of dupilumab in treating ACD is still in the early phases of investigation. One case series of 2 patients with severe, refractory ACD showed promising results. Although ACD is not classically considered a Th2-mediated condition, dupilumab anecdotally reduced severe pruritus and diminished the need for topical betamethasone dipropionate and tacrolimus in these patients.[57] Further study is required to employ dupilumab as an approved ACD therapy, but off-label use may be a possibility for patients suffering from refractory ACD symptoms.

When evaluated for its safety profile, dupilumab was noted to have serious adverse events in 4% of patients who received the therapy at 2-week intervals. The most common adverse reactions over the 52-week trial were injection site reactions (15%) and conjunctivitis (14%).[58] A multicenter open-label extension study evaluating patients from 12 phase 1, phase 2, and phase 3 trials assessing for long-term safety noted that most patients experienced a mild-to-moderate adverse effect (70.7%), while only 5.0% of patients experienced a serious adverse event, such as squamous cell carcinoma of the skin, osteoarthritis, ligament rupture, depression, and worsening of AD; no deaths were reported with patients taking dupilumab, and only 1.8% of patients experienced an adverse event that required permanent discontinuation of the drug.[53] Of note, dupilumab is not thought to cause significant labortory abnormalities and therefore does not require initial or ongoing laboratory monitoring during therapy. Overall, current research seems to indicate that dupilumab is a safe and effective option for the treatment of moderate-to severe AD. Other monoclonal antibodies have been developed that target the IL-4 and IL-13 cytokines themselves, such as pascolizumab, lebrikizumab, and tralokinumab. Both lebrikizumab and tralokinumab are currently being studied for AD.[59]

## JANUS KINASE INHIBITORS IN ATOPIC DERMATITIS

JAK inhibitors present another immunomodulatory route through which the inflammation in AD can be suppressed. Janus kinase (JAK) includes a family of 4 nonreceptor tyrosine kinases (JAK1-3, TYK2) that work in conjunction with the signal transducer and activators of transcription (STAT) family of proteins to form the JAK-STAT pathway. This pathway is essential for driving the function of immune cells, including the B-, T-, NK-, and mast cell lines. Inhibition of the JAK-STAT pathway has shown promise for various inflammatory conditions, including AD.[60] Numerous JAK inhibitors are available or are the subject of active research, each of which is selective for a respective set of JAK homologs, including: tofacitinib, ruxolitinib, abrocitinib, upada-citinib, baricitinib, filgotinib, and gusacitinib, and others still in development. The anti-inflammatory effects of JAK inhibitors tend to have a rapid onset of effect in the treatment of pruritus in AD relative to that of biologic therapies. Although some have speculated the anti-inflammatory effects of JAK inhibitors may be helpful for ACD (Cinats, and colleagues, 2018), there are currently no studies investigating the efficacy of JAK inhibitors in the treatment of ACD.

Numerous randomized-controlled trials have investigated the use of JAK inhibitors in AD. Two percent topical formulations of tofacitinib were found to lead to a 81.7% reduction in baseline EASI score versus 29.9% reduction with vehicle ointment after 4 weeks in a study of 69 patients (P<.001).[61] Topical 1.5% ruxolitinib twice daily led to an improvement of EASI score by 71.6% versus 15.5% improvement seen with vehicle control in a study of 307 patients; incremental improvements were seen as lower dose groups were transitioned to 1.5% ruxolitinib twice daily.[62] Oral abrocitinib 200 mg and 100 mg doses were associated with clear or almost clear investigator global assessment (IGA) responses in 44% and 24% of patients, respectively, versus 8% in control groups (P<.001 and P=.0037, respectively). The 200 mg group had 63% of patients achieve 75% reduction in EASI score, while 40% achieved the same improvement with 100 mg dosing (vs 12% in control group, P<.0001).[63] Sixty-one percent of patients taking oral baricitinib 4 mg achieved EASI 50% reduction versus 37% with control (P=.027) at 16 weeks, with a notably higher rate of adverse effects in the 4 mg baricitinib group (71% vs 49% of control group).[64] Many clinical trials for the treatment of AD with JAK inhibitors have been conducted or are currently under-way for tofacitinib, ruxolitinib, abrocitinib, upadacitinib, and baricitinib.[65]

Concerns over patient safety and laboratory monitoring may limit adoption of JAK inhibitors, particularly higher-strength oral formulations. The higher-dose regimen (10 mg twice daily) of oral tofacitinib was given a black box warning by the FDA in 2019 for an increased risk of deep venous thrombosis, pulmonary embolism, and death[66]; a similar label has been given to other JAK inhibitors, including upadacitinib. These safety concerns may limit the broader use of oral JAK inhibitors for AD, but must be weighed in context with potentially superior efficacy and a favorable oral route of administration. The risk-to-benefit ratio may differ for topical JAK inhibitor formula-tions, such as ruxolitinib, for which a clinical trial for the treatment of AD is underway. Currently, the role of oral and topical JAK inhibitors for AD is not yet fully defined, and remains an area of active research.

## PHOSPHODIESTERASE INHIBITORS

Phosphodiesterase (PDE) inhibitors are another anti-inflammatory route that has been studied for the treatment of AD. Chief among the PDE family is PDE4, whose inhibition has been shown to decrease production of numerous proinflammatory cytokines, such as tumor necrosis factor-alpha (TNF-alpha), IL-2, IL-12, and IL-23.[67] Crisaborole is a major example of a PDE4 inhibitor, which was approved for the topical treatment of mild-to-moderate AD in 2016. Other PDE inhibitors have been trialed for the treat-ment of AD. Apremilast is another PDE4 inhibitor that has been studied in a phase 2 randomized-controlled trial. This trial demonstrated that 40 mg twice daily dosing of apremilast was associated with a 31.6% reduction in EASI score versus an 11.0% reduction in control patients (P=.04); an increased rate of adverse events (including 6 cases of cellulitis) was noted in the 40 mg twice daily treatment group, requiring in-vestigators to halt this treatment group.[68] Apremilast has proven more efficacious in the treatment of psoriasis. In conjunction with the availability of more favorable

| Table 1 Selected translational advances | | |
|---|---|---|
| **Pathomechanism** | **Potential Target** | **Potential Therapy** |
| Impaired skin barrier | Ceramide deficiency | Specialized moisturizers |
| Dysbiosis | S. aureus overgrowth | Probiotics |
| Inflammation | IL-4, IL-13, others JAK-STAT pathway PDE | Anti-receptor and anti-cytokine antibodies Topical and oral JAK inhibitors PDE inhibitors |
| Itch | IL-31 | Anti-IL-31 antibody |

*Abbreviations:* JAK-STAT, Janus Kinase and Signal Transducer and Activators of Transcription; PDE, phosphodiesterase; S, aureus, Staphylococcus areus.

alternatives, there has been less interest in the continued study of apremilast for the treatment of AD.

The treatment of ACD with PDE inhibitors has seen much less study. A small investigation of 5 patients with recalcitrant ACD treated with 20 mg of apremilast twice daily demonstrated a mean reduction in EASI score by 42% ($P=.026$), with a relatively lower starting average starting EASI score of 12.5 versus AD patients included in this study (Volf and colleagues, 2012). Despite results indicating possible efficacy of apremilast in treating ACD, no further studies have been conducted; no other PDE inhibitors, including crisaborole, have been studied for the treatment of ACD.

## NEW THERAPEUTIC APPROACHES FOR DERMATITIS

Recent efforts in personalized, precision therapy warrant new and innovative methods of symptom control and targeting underlying pathologic processes. As the growing number of players in AD pathophysiology are found and understood, one drifts further from the idea that AD and ACD are single diseases with broad therapeutic approaches. From interrupting the inflammatory pathway to bolstering the skin barrier, numerous promising therapies are in the pipeline.

Despite advances in target-specific anti-inflammatory biologic agents for severe dermatitis, a holistic approach to the topical treatment of dermatitis and rehabilitation of the skin's barrier function at a cellular level continues to fall short for some patients. Although there are numerous ways to optimize the skin barrier, some studies have suggested doing so by correcting the sphingolipid profile of inflammatory skin in AD. With greater understanding about the precise role of lysosomes and the pathologic disruption of ceramide metabolism comes the possibility of pathogenesis-targeted topical therapies rather than simply symptomatic ones. A recent study fortified this concept with an off-label regimen including amitriptyline (in an antiapoptotic role) and linoleic acid (for lysosomal protection and ceramide synthesis stabilization) completely, clearing lesions after 60 days of use. Patients also had sustained results with frequent application of prophylactic linoleic acid cream.[69] **(Table 1)**.

## SUMMARY

Much remains unknown about the pathophysiology of dermatitis, but a better understanding is being gleaned from advances in the underlying pathogenesis bearing fruit with therapeutic hopefuls seen in clinical trials, enabling the virtuous cycle of translational medicine. Many facets of the immunobiology of dermatitis have been uncovered as more inflammatory targets are successfully exploited in the treatment of dermatitis. Such treatment options are beginning to make their way into clinical practice, including biologic agents such as dupilumab and small molecule agents such as the JAK inhibitors.

As the armamentarium of therapies for dermatitis continues to grow, and excitement builds around novel approaches to treatment, clinicians must draw on their experiences with decades of well-founded therapies and newer, more ambitious routes to optimize care for patients. In so doing, the march toward precision medicine will continue in earnest.

## CLINICS CARE POINTS

- Regardless of the initiating factor, skin barrier dysfunction is central to AD and should be a primary treatment consideration.
- Treating the inflammation of AD generally also improves itch, as many of the mediators are shared.
- The treat to target for atopic dermatitis continues to rise as there are newer and more powerful therapies available, and keeping the skin clear safely and comfortably is now possible for many patients.

## DISCLOSURE

Dr P. Lio reports research grants/funding from the National Eczema Association, Regeneron/Sanofi Genzyme, and AbbVie; is on the speaker's bureau for Regeneron/Sanofi Genzyme, Pfizer, Galderma, and L'Oreal; reports consulting/advisory boards for Dermavant, Regeneron/Sanofi Genzyme, Dermira, Pfizer, LEO Pharmaceuticals, AbbVie, Kiniksa, Eli Lilly, Micreos (stock options), L'Oreal, Pierre-Fabre, Johnson & Johnson, Level Ex, Unilever, Menlo Therapeutics, Theraplex, IntraDerm, Exeltis, AOBiome, United States. Realm Therapeutics, Altus Labs (stock options), Galderma, Verrica, Arbonne, Amyris, Bodewell, and Burt's Bees. In addition, Dr P. Lio has a patent pending for a Theraplex product with royalties paid and is a Board member and Scientific Advisory Committee Member of the National Eczema Association and an investor at LearnSkin. The other authors report no conflicts.

## REFERENCES

1. About Translation. 2017. Available at: https://ncats.nih.gov/translation. Accessed October 29, 2020.
2. Schlapbach C, Navarini AA. The continuing evolution of targeted therapy for inflammatory skin disease. Semin Immunopathol 2016;38(1):123–33.
3. Lohman ME, Lio PA. Comparison of psoriasis and atopic dermatitis guidelines—an argument for aggressive atopic dermatitis management. Pediatr Dermatol 2017;34(6):739–42. Available at: https://onlinelibrary.wiley.com/doi/abs/10.1111/pde.13282.
4. Williams HC. Epidemiology of human atopic dermatitis–seven areas of notable progress and seven areas of notable ignorance. Vet Dermatol 2013;24(1):3.e2.
5. Kim BE, Leung DYM, Boguniewicz M, et al. Loricrin and involucrin expression is down-regulated by Th2 cytokines through STAT-6. Clin Immunol 2008;126(3):332–7.
6. Strugar TL, Kuo A, Seité S, et al. Connecting the dots: from skin barrier dysfunction to allergic sensitization, and the role of moisturizers in repairing the skin barrier. J Drugs Dermatol 2019;18(6):581.

7. Brown SJ, McLean WHI. One remarkable molecule: filaggrin. J Invest Dermatol 2012;132(3 Pt 2):751–62.

8. Dennin M, Lio PA. Filaggrin and childhood eczema. Arch Dis Child 2017;102(12): 1101–2.

9. Eichenfield LF, Tom WL, Berger TG, et al. Guidelines of care for the management of atopic dermatitis: section 2. Management and treatment of atopic dermatitis with topical therapies. J Am Acad Dermatol 2014;71(1):116–32.

10. Shi VY, Tran K, Lio PA. A comparison of physicochemical properties of a selection of modern moisturizers: hydrophilic index and pH. J Drugs Dermatol 2012;11(5): 633–6.

11. van Zuuren EJ, Fedorowicz Z, Christensen R, et al. Emollients and moisturisers for eczema. Cochrane Database Syst Rev 2017;2017(2). CD012119 Available at: https://www.ncbi.nlm.nih.gov/pmc/articles/pmc6464068/.

12. Simpson EL, Chalmers JR, Hanifin JM, et al. Emollient enhancement of the skin barrier from birth offers effective atopic dermatitis prevention. J Allergy Clin Immunol 2014;134(4):818–23.

13. Chalmers JR, Haines RH, Bradshaw LE, et al. Daily emollient during infancy for prevention of eczema: the BEEP randomised controlled trial. Lancet 2020. https://doi.org/10.1016/S0140-6736(19)32984-8.

14. Skjerven HO, Rehbinder EM, Vettukattil R, et al. Skin emollient and early complementary feeding to prevent infant atopic dermatitis (PreventADALL): a factorial, multicentre, cluster-randomised trial. Lancet 2020;395(10228):951–61.

15. Lowe AJ, Su JC, Allen KJ, et al. A randomized trial of a barrier lipid replacement strategy for the prevention of atopic dermatitis and allergic sensitization: the PEBBLES pilot study. Br J Dermatol 2018;178(1):e19–21.

16. Bantz SK, Zhu Z, Zheng T. The atopic march: progression from atopic dermatitis to allergic rhinitis and asthma. J Clin Cell Immunol 2014;5(2). https://doi.org/10.4172/2155-9899.1000202.

17. Natsume O, Ohya Y. Recent advancement to prevent the development of allergy and allergic diseases and therapeutic strategy in the perspective of barrier dysfunction. Allergol Int 2018;67(1):24–31.

18. Hepburn L, Hijnen DJ, Sellman BR, et al. The complex biology and contribution of Staphylococcus aureus in atopic dermatitis, current and future therapies. Br J Dermatol 2017;177(1):63–71.

19. Cho SH, Strickland I, Tomkinson A, et al. Preferential binding of Staphylococcus aureus to skin sites of Th2-mediated inflammation in a murine model. J Invest Dermatol 2001;116(5):658–63.

20. Spaulding A, Satterwhite E, Lin Y-C, et al. Comparison of Staphylococcus aureus strains for ability to cause infective endocarditis and lethal sepsis in rabbits. Front Cell Infect Microbiol 2012;2:18.

21. Al Kindi A, Williams H, Matsuda K, et al. Staphylococcus aureus second immunoglobulin-binding protein drives atopic dermatitis via IL-33. J Allergy Clin Immunol 2020. https://doi.org/10.1016/j.jaci.2020.09.023.

22. Krasteva M, Kehren J, Horand F, et al. Dual role of dendritic cells in the induction and down-regulation of antigen-specific cutaneous inflammation. J Immunol 1998;160(3):1181–90.

23. Raffi J, Suresh R, Botto N, et al. The impact of dupilumab on patch testing and the prevalence of comorbid allergic contact dermatitis in recalcitrant atopic dermatitis: a retrospective chart review. J Am Acad Dermatol 2020;82(1):132–8.

24. Huang JT, Abrams M, Tlougan B, et al. Treatment of Staphylococcus aureus colonization in atopic dermatitis decreases disease severity. Pediatrics 2009;123(5): e808–14.

25. Leung TH, Zhang LF, Wang J, et al. Topical hypochlorite ameliorates NF-κB-mediated skin diseases in mice. J Clin Invest 2013;123(12):5361–70.

26. Perez-Nazario N, Yoshida T, Fridy S, et al. Bleach baths significantly reduce itch and severity of atopic dermatitis with no significant change in S. aureus colonization and only modest effects on skin barrier function. J Invest Dermatol 2015; 135:s37.

27. Sawada Y, Tong Y, Barangi M, et al. Dilute bleach baths used for treatment of atopic dermatitis are not antimicrobial in vitro. J Allergy Clin Immunol 2019; 143(5):1946–8.

28. Hon KL, Tsang YCK, Lee VWY, et al. Efficacy of sodium hypochlorite (bleach) baths to reduce Staphylococcus aureus colonization in childhood onset moderate-to-severe eczema: A randomized, placebo-controlled cross-over trial. J Dermatolog Treat 2016;27(2):156–62.

29. Gonzalez ME, Schaffer JV, Orlow SJ, et al. Cutaneous microbiome effects of fluticasone propionate cream and adjunctive bleach baths in childhood atopic dermatitis. J Am Acad Dermatol 2016;75(3):481–93.e8.

30. Scharschmidt TC, Vasquez KS, Truong H-A, et al. A wave of regulatory t cells into neonatal skin mediates tolerance to commensal microbes. Immunity 2015;43(5): 1011–21.

31. Myles IA, Castillo CR, Barbian KD, et al. Therapeutic responses to Roseomonas mucosa in atopic dermatitis may involve lipid-mediated TNF-related epithelial repair. Sci Transl Med 2020;12(560). https://doi.org/10.1126/scitranslmed. aaz8631.

32. Hamid Q, Boguniewicz M, Leung DY. Differential in situ cytokine gene expression in acute versus chronic atopic dermatitis. J Clin Invest 1994;94(2):870–6.

33. Czarnowicki T, Krueger JG, Guttman-Yassky E. Skin barrier and immune dysregulation in atopic dermatitis: an evolving story with important clinical implications. J Allergy Clin Immunol Pract 2014;2(4):371–9 [quiz: 380–1].

34. Brunner PM, Guttman-Yassky E, Leung DYM. The immunology of atopic dermatitis and its reversibility with broad-spectrum and targeted therapies. J Allergy Clin Immunol 2017;139(4S):S65–76.

35. Reinhold U, Liu L, Sesterhenn J, et al. The CD7- T cell subset represents the majority of IL-5-secreting cells within CD4+CD45RA- T cells. Clin Exp Immunol 1996; 106(3):555–9.

36. Spergel JM, Mizoguchi E, Oettgen H, et al. Roles of TH1 and TH2 cytokines in a murine model of allergic dermatitis. J Clin Invest 1999;103(8):1103–11.

37. Leckie MJ, ten Brinke A, Khan J, et al. Effects of an interleukin-5 blocking monoclonal antibody on eosinophils, airway hyper-responsiveness, and the late asthmatic response. Lancet 2000;356(9248):2144–8.

38. Oldhoff JM, Darsow U, Werfel T, et al. Anti-IL-5 recombinant humanized monoclonal antibody (mepolizumab) for the treatment of atopic dermatitis. Allergy 2005;60(5):693–6.

39. Kang EG, Narayana PK, Pouliquen IJ, et al. Efficacy and safety of mepolizumab administered subcutaneously for moderate to severe atopic dermatitis. Allergy 2019. https://doi.org/10.1111/all.14050.

40. Corren J. Anti-interleukin-5 antibody therapy in asthma and allergies. Curr Opin Allergy Clin Immunol 2011;11(6):565–70.

41. Dillon SR, Sprecher C, Hammond A, et al. Interleukin 31, a cytokine produced by activated T cells, induces dermatitis in mice. Nat Immunol 2004;5(7):752–60.
42. Raap U, Wichmann K, Bruder M, et al. Correlation of IL-31 serum levels with severity of atopic dermatitis. J Allergy Clin Immunol 2008;122(2):421–3.
43. Ezzat MHM, Hasan ZE, Shaheen KYA. Serum measurement of interleukin-31 (IL-31) in paediatric atopic dermatitis: elevated levels correlate with severity scoring. J Eur Acad Dermatol Venereol 2011;25(3):334–9.
44. Cornelissen C, Lüscher-Firzlaff J, Baron JM, et al. Signaling by IL-31 and functional consequences. Eur J Cell Biol 2012;91(6–7):552–66.
45. Cornelissen C, Marquardt Y, Czaja K, et al. IL-31 regulates differentiation and filaggrin expression in human organotypic skin models. J Allergy Clin Immunol 2012;129(2):426–33, 433.e1-e8.
46. Neis MM, Peters B, Dreuw A, et al. Enhanced expression levels of IL-31 correlate with IL-4 and IL-13 in atopic and allergic contact dermatitis. J Allergy Clin Immunol 2006;118(4):930–7.
47. Silverberg JI, Pinter A, Pulka G, et al. Phase 2B randomized study of nemolizumab in adults with moderate-to-severe atopic dermatitis and severe pruritus. J Allergy Clin Immunol 2020;145(1):173–82.
48. Petronelli M. Breakthrough therapy designation granted to nemolizumab for pruritus. Dermatol Times 2020;41(1). Available at: https://www.dermatologytimes.com/biologics/breakthrough-therapy-designation-granted-nemolizumab-pruritus.
49. Seltmann J, Werfel T, Wittmann M. Evidence for a regulatory loop between IFN-γ and IL-33 in skin inflammation. Exp Dermatol 2013;22(2):102–7.
50. AnaptysBio Reports Etokimab ATLAS phase 2b clinical trial in moderate-to-severe atopic dermatitis fails to meet primary endpoint. Available at: https://ir.anaptysbio.com/news-releases/news-release-details/anaptysbio-reports-etokimab-atlas-phase-2b-clinical-trial. Accessed November 1, 2020.
51. Brandt EB, Sivaprasad U. Th2 Cytokines and atopic dermatitis. J Clin Cell Immunol 2011;2(3). https://doi.org/10.4172/2155-9899.1000110.
52. Tazawa T, Sugiura H, Sugiura Y, et al. Relative importance of IL-4 and IL-13 in lesional skin of atopic dermatitis. Arch Dermatol Res 2004;295(11):459–64.
53. Deleuran M, Thaçi D, Beck LA, et al. Dupilumab shows long-term safety and efficacy in patients with moderate to severe atopic dermatitis enrolled in a phase 3 open-label extension study. J Am Acad Dermatol 2020;82(2):377–88.
54. Simpson EL, Bieber T, Guttman-Yassky E, et al. Two phase 3 trials of dupilumab versus placebo in atopic dermatitis. N Engl J Med 2016;375(24):2335–48.
55. Cork MJ, Thaçi D, Eichenfield LF, et al. Dupilumab in adolescents with uncontrolled moderate-to-severe atopic dermatitis: results from a phase IIa open-label trial and subsequent phase III open-label extension. Br J Dermatol 2020; 182(1):85–96.
56. Sanofi. FDA approves Dupixent (dupilumab) as first biologic medicine for children aged 6 to 11 years with moderate-to-severe atopic dermatitis. 2020. Available at: https://www.sanofi.com/en/media-room/press-releases/2020/2020-05-26-17-40-00. Accessed May 14, 2021
57. Chipalkatti N, Lee N, Zancanaro P, et al. A retrospective review of dupilumab for atopic dermatitis patients with allergic contact dermatitis. J Am Acad Dermatol 2019;80(4):1166–7.
58. Blauvelt A, de Bruin-Weller M, Gooderham M, et al. Long-term management of moderate-to-severe atopic dermatitis with dupilumab and concomitant topical corticosteroids (LIBERTY AD CHRONOS): a 1-year, randomised, double-blinded, placebo-controlled, phase 3 trial. Lancet 2017;389(10086):2287–303.

59. Deleanu D, Nedelea I. Biological therapies for atopic dermatitis: an update. Exp Ther Med 2019;17(2):1061–7.
60. Tegtmeyer K, Zhao J, Maloney NJ, et al. Off-label studies on tofacitinib in dermatology: a review. J Dermatolog Treat 2019;1–11. https://doi.org/10.1080/09546634.2019.1673877.
61. Bissonnette R, Papp KA, Poulin Y, et al. Topical tofacitinib for atopic dermatitis: a phase IIa randomized trial. Br J Dermatol 2016;175(5):902–11.
62. Kim BS, Howell MD, Sun K, et al. Treatment of atopic dermatitis with ruxolitinib cream (JAK1/JAK2 inhibitor) or triamcinolone cream. J Allergy Clin Immunol 2020;145(2):572–82.
63. Simpson EL, Sinclair R, Forman S, et al. Efficacy and safety of abrocitinib in adults and adolescents with moderate-to-severe atopic dermatitis (JADE MONO-1): a multicentre, double-blind, randomised, placebo-controlled, phase 3 trial. Lancet 2020;396(10246):255–66.
64. Guttman-Yassky E, Silverberg JI, Nemoto O, et al. Baricitinib in adult patients with moderate-to-severe atopic dermatitis: a phase 2 parallel, double-blinded, randomized placebo-controlled multiple-dose study. J Am Acad Dermatol 2019; 80(4):913–21.e9.
65. Home - ClinicalTrials.gov. Available at: https://clinicaltrials.gov/. Accessed November 1, 2020.
66. Communication FDS. FDA approves boxed warning about increased risk of blood clots and death with higher dose of arthritis and ulcerative colitis medicine tofacitinib (Xeljanz, Xeljanz XR). U.S. Food & Drug Administration. 2019. Available at: https://www.fda.gov/drugs/drug-safety-and-availability/fda-approves-boxed-warning-about-increased-risk-blood-clots-and-death-higher-dose-arthritis-and. Accessed May 14, 2021.
67. Maloney NJ, Zhao J, Tegtmeyer K, et al. Off-label studies on apremilast in dermatology: a review. J Dermatolog Treat 2020;31(2):131–40.
68. Simpson EL, Imafuku S, Poulin Y, et al. A phase 2 randomized trial of apremilast in patients with atopic dermatitis. J Invest Dermatol 2019;139(5):1063–72.
69. Blaess M, Wenzel F, Csuk R, et al. Topical use of amitriptyline and linoleic acid to restore ceramide rheostat in atopic dermatitis lesions - a case report. Pharmazie 2019;74(9):563–5.

# Environmental Causes of Dermatitis

Jannett Nguyen, MD, Jennifer K. Chen, MD*

## KEYWORDS

- Allergic contact dermatitis • Environmental dermatitis • Exogenous dermatitis
- Regional dermatitis • Skin allergens

## KEY POINTS

- Rash morphology can help distinguish between exogenous and endogenous causes of dermatitis. Asymmetry, geometric shape, and linearity may suggest exogenous causes.
- Allergy to metals, such as nickel and cobalt, is frequent. Other common contact allergens are preservatives, emollients, fragrances, and dyes found in personal care, cosmetic, and household products.
- Rash distribution is helpful in suggesting potential culprit allergens.
- Patch testing is needed to confirm contact allergy.

## INTRODUCTION

Exogenous dermatitis is triggered by environmental irritants and allergens, which account for 80% and 20% of contact dermatitis cases, respectively. Irritant contact dermatitis (ICD) is caused by direct cytotoxic effect; in contrast, allergic contact dermatitis (ACD) is caused by a type IV delayed hypersensitivity reaction that requires prior hapten sensitization.[1] These diagnoses are not mutually exclusive, and it is common for the causes of contact dermatitis to be multifactorial. Failure to diagnose contact dermatitis may result in overlooking a potentially curable driver of disease.

## DISCUSSION
### Exogenous Versus Endogenous Dermatitis

Both exogenous and endogenous causes of dermatitis can result in erythema and vesicle or bulla formation in acute stages, and scaling, lichenification, and fissuring in chronic stages. However, there are clinical features that are more suggestive of exogenous rather than endogenous dermatitis (**Box 1**).[2,3] Morphology is helpful: exogeneous dermatitis is classically a well-demarcated, erythematous, vesicular, or scaly

Department of Dermatology, Stanford University School of Medicine, 450 Broadway Street, Pavilion C, 2nd Floor, Redwood City, CA 94063, USA
* Corresponding author.
E-mail address: jenniferkchen@stanford.edu

Immunol Allergy Clin N Am 41 (2021) 375–392
https://doi.org/10.1016/j.iac.2021.04.002
0889-8561/21/© 2021 Elsevier Inc. All rights reserved.
immunology.theclinics.com

> **Box 1**
> **Clinical clues suggestive of exogenous causes of dermatitis**
>
> - Sharp demarcation
> - Asymmetry
> - Geometric shape
> - Linear arrangement
> - Distribution atypical for a known endogenous dermatosis (eg, genital involvement in atopic dermatitis; airborne distribution)
> - Sudden worsening or change in distribution of dermatitis

patch or plaque involving the area of contact. Other morphologic clues include asymmetry (although symmetric ACD is also common), geometric shape (**Fig. 1**), and linearity (**Fig. 2**).

Dermatitis distribution can provide additional support for a possible exogenous cause. Any distribution that is changing or atypical for known endogenous dermatoses (eg, genital involvement in atopic dermatitis) increases the likelihood of contact dermatitis. Examples of other high-yield ACD distributions include airborne and photodistributions. Both involve the face and neck, with a sharp cutoff at the V of the neck corresponding to clothing; however, the former tends to spare the central face, whereas the latter spares sun-protected areas, such as the eyelid creases, neck folds, and postauricular or submental regions.[1,4]

### Allergic Contact Dermatitis and Irritant Contact Dermatitis

Clinical features can help distinguish between ACD and ICD. Absence of itch generally argues against ACD, which is typically characterized by at least moderate pruritus. In contrast, ICD is often associated with burning, stinging, and pain, and itch may be

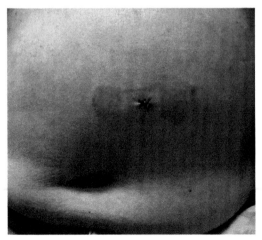

**Fig. 1.** Irritant contact dermatitis from a bandage applied to the abdomen following skin biopsy. Note the rectangular erythematous patch corresponding to areas of contact with adhesive.

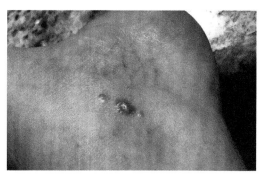

**Fig. 2.** Allergic contact dermatitis from poison oak after hiking. Note the linearly arranged erythematous vesicles corresponding to where a leaf brushed against the ankle.

absent or mild to moderate. ACD is more likely to spread, whereas ICD tends to remain limited to the area of exposure.[5] Additionally, ACD tends to occur in a delayed fashion at least 24 hours after exposure, whereas ICD tends to occur within 24 hours.

The gold standard for diagnosing ACD is the combination of relevant clinical presentation (ie, history of exposure), patch testing, and demonstration of rash resolution with avoidance of identified allergens.[2,6,7] In contrast, there is no commonly used test to diagnose ICD, and it is often diagnosed based on history and temporal course, or by exclusion following negative patch testing. Any given contactant may have irritant properties, allergenic properties, or both. Frequent causes of ICD include wet work (eg, water), bodily fluids (eg, saliva from lip licking or drooling, irritant diaper dermatitis in babies, urinary or fecal incontinence in the elderly), detergents/cleansers, solvents, glues, acid and alkali chemicals, cutting oils, metal salts, and disinfectants.[8] In comparison, common culprit allergens for ACD include metals, preservatives, fragrance, surfactants, emollients, and dyes found in jewelry, clothing, personal care products, or household cleaning agents.

ACD affects about 4.5 million people in North America annually and can cause significant morbidity.[9] The identification of causative allergens and implementation of allergen avoidance can lead to disease remission and improve quality of life.[9] The remainder of this review focuses on common causes of ACD, and how dermatitis distribution is suggestive of particular culprit allergens. Patch testing is required to confirm the causative allergens.

### Overview of Common Contact Allergens

The most common contact allergens in North America have recently been reported to include nickel, methylisothiazolinone (MI), methylchloroisothiazolinone/MI (Kathon CG, MCI/MI), fragrance mix (I and II), formaldehyde, balsam of Peru, neomycin, bacitracin, para-phenylenediamine (PPD), cobalt, carba mix, lanolin alcohol, and propylene glycol.[10] **Table 1** summarizes these and other notable allergens, and their associated sources of exposure. The most common contact allergens are further discussed next.

Nickel and cobalt are common metal allergens, and nickel has remained the most commonly reported allergen in patch-tested patients for decades.[10] Nickel is a strong metal often incorporated into metal alloys used for machine parts and equipment. Personal items, such as jewelry, watches, and clothing fasteners, and household items, such as coins, keys, scissors, and batteries, commonly contain nickel. It has been hypothesized that high rates of nickel allergy could be attributable to ear piercing,

**Table 1**
**Prevalent allergens and common sources of exposure**

| Allergen | Common Sources of Allergen Exposure |
|---|---|
| *Preservatives* | |
| Methylisothiazolinone[a]<br>Kathon CG, MCI/MI[a]<br>Iodopropynyl<br>  butylcarbamate<br>Parabens<br>Formaldehyde[a] releasing<br>  preservatives<br>  Quaternium-15<br>  2-bromo-2-nitropropane-1,3-diol<br>  Diazolidinyl urea<br>  Imidazolidinyl urea<br>  DMDM hydantoin | Cosmetics, personal care products, toiletries, household cleaning agents, metalworking fluids, wipes, glues, printing ink |
| *Emulsifiers* | |
| Propylene glycol[a]<br>Oleamidopropyl<br>  dimethylamine | Cosmetics, personal care products, topical medicaments, saline solution, baby wipes, paint, automotive care |
| *Surfactants* | |
| Cocamidopropyl betaine | Shampoos, soaps, cosmetics, toothpaste |
| *Emollients* | |
| Lanolin[a] | Personal care products, moisturizing ointments/creams, medicaments |
| *Fragrance/flavoring agents* | |
| Fragrance/botanicals:<br>  Fragrance mix I[a]<br>  Fragrance mix II[a]<br>  Balsam of Peru<br>    (*Myroxylon pereirae*)[a]<br>  Hydroperoxides of limonene<br>  Hydroperoxides of linalool<br>  Tea tree oil | Perfume, cosmetics, personal care products, household products, facial tissue, air freshener, medicaments, wax/polishes, paints, metalworking fluids |
| Flavor:<br>  Cinnamic aldehyde<br>  Carvone<br>  Menthol | Toothpaste, mouthwash, cosmetics, cooking and baking flavorings, chewing gum, medication |
| *Dyes* | |
| p-Phenylenediamine[a] | Permanent hair dye, hair rinse, black henna, textile dye, shampoo-in highlight, printing ink |
| Disperse blue 106/124 | Textile dye (synthetic blends) |
| *Rubber*<br>  *accelerators/antioxidants* | |
| Carba mix[a]<br>Mercaptobenzothiazole<br>Mercapto mix<br>Thiuram mix | Rubber products, gloves, rubber shoes and insoles, sponge makeup applicators, medical equipment, elastics in clothing, fungicide/insecticide |
| Mixed dialkyl thioureas | Neoprene, athletic shoe insoles, photocopy, photography |

(*continued on next page*)

**Table 1**
**(continued)**

| Allergen | Common Sources of Allergen Exposure |
|---|---|
| Black rubber mix | Black or gray rubber products (eg, tires, sporting equipment) |
| *Metals* | |
| Nickel[a] Cobalt[a] Gold sodium thiosulfate | Jewelry, keys, clothing fasteners, machinery, cutting fluids, medical devices, tools/equipment, ceramics, paint |
| *Plastics/glues* | |
| Acrylates | Artificial nails, nail glues, surgical glues, bone cement, dental materials, hygiene pads, hearing aids, contact lenses, eyeglasses, printing inks, plastics, paint |
| Colophony | Resin/rosin, adhesive, plastics, modeling clay, medication, printing ink, cosmetics, wax, glossy paper |
| Epoxy resin | Adhesive, plastics, paints, electrical insulation, dental bonding agents, protective coatings, vinyl gloves, polyvinyl chloride |
| p-tert-butylphenol formaldehyde resin | Adhesive used with neoprene, shoes, others |
| *Medicaments* | |
| Neomycin[a] Bacitracin[a] | Antibiotic ointment/creams and solutions, antibiotic irrigation fluid, bandages |
| Budesonide Tixocortol-21-pivalate | Corticosteroid medications |
| Benzocaine | Anesthetic topical ointments/creams, cough drops, sore throat sprays, antibacterial washes |
| Ethylenediamine dihydrochloride | Antihistamine topical ointments/creams, epoxy resin hardener, insecticide, fungicide, electroplating |
| *Plants* | |
| Urushiol | Poison oak, poison ivy, poison sumac |
| Sesquiterpene lactones (Compositae mix) | *Asteraceae* plants (eg, chrysanthemum, feverfew, arnica), personal care products with botanic extracts |
| Tulipalin | Tulips, Peruvian lilies |
| *Other* | |
| Ethyleneurea/melamine formaldehyde resin | Permanent press clothing |
| Glyceryl thioglycolate | Permanent hair wave solutions |
| α-Tocopherol | Synthetic vitamin E ointments/creams |
| Tosylamide formaldehyde resin | Nail polishes/hardeners |

[a] Indicates top 15 most common allergens per recent North American Contact Dermatitis Group patch test results.[10]

wherein nickel-containing metal posts have direct contact with injured (ie, pierced) skin.[1,11,12] Like nickel, cobalt is also used in metal alloys. Cobalt is found in bricks, cement, cobalt-based pigments, and metal tools and utensils. Because cobalt is often combined with other metals, about 80% of those with cobalt allergy are cosensitized to nickel or chromium.[1,12]

MCI and MI are preservatives frequently used in household and personal care products, in combination and in the form of MI by itself. Currently, MI is the most common preservative allergen and second most common allergen overall in North America,[10] and may be found in laundry, dish, and cleaning products, and hair products, hand sanitizers, moisturizers, sunscreens, and other personal care products.[13] Historically, use of sanitary wet wipes has been heavily associated with sensitization to MI,[14] although currently most wet wipes no longer contain MI. Rates of sensitivity to MCI/MI and MI have increased dramatically in recent years, with regulatory changes occurring in 2005 that allowed for higher concentrations of MI (100 ppm, previously <3.75 ppm) in consumer products likely playing a large contributory role.[12,15] Of note, it is critical to patch test to MI alone (typically tested at 2000 ppm), because patch testing to MCI/MI misses around half of cases of contact allergy to MI alone.[16]

Another common allergen with preservative properties is formaldehyde, an ubiquitous colorless gas. In modern society, formaldehyde itself is rarely used in personal care products. Thus, positive patch testing to formaldehyde usually indicates allergy to formaldehyde-releasing preservatives found in industrial and household products, and less frequently formaldehyde resins used in fabric finishers for wrinkle-resistant clothing, or tosylamide formaldehyde resin added to nail hardeners or polish to help polish adhere to the nail and strengthen the coating.[1,12,17] The presence of formaldehyde has been recently identified in 8.6% of personal care products without formaldehyde in their ingredient lists, underscoring the challenges in avoiding this ubiquitous allergen.[18]

Fragrances are another example of ubiquitous allergens, incorporated into most personal care and household products to add scent or to mask unpleasant scent. Fragrance mix I and II are commonly used in patch testing to identify fragrance allergy,[1,12,19] along with balsam of Peru, a fragrant liquid harvested from *Myroxylon balsamum var. pereirae* trees. A positive patch test to the latter may also indicate allergy to clove, cinnamon, Jamaican pepper, cola, tobacco, wine, or vermouth.[1,12] Patients with fragrance allergy should be directed to search for "fragrance-free products," rather than "unscented" products, which may contain a masking fragrance to cancel out odor.

The most common medicament contact allergens are neomycin and bacitracin, topical antibiotics found in prescription and over-the-counter preparations, such as first-aid kits, hemorrhoid creams, and otic and ophthalmic solutions.[20,21] Although they have different chemical structures, cosensitization to neomycin and bacitracin is frequently observed, because they are often used together in preparations, such as Neosporin (Johnson & Johnson, New Brunswick, New Jersey).[1]

Rubber accelerators used in manufacturing rubber products (eg, gloves, goggles, rubber bands, and sports equipment) are allergenic, the most common being carba mix.[12] Pesticides and fungicides may also contain carba mix. Other rubber allergens include mercapto mix, thiuram mix, mixed dialkyl thioureas, and black rubber mix.[1,12]

Propylene glycol is a preservative, emulsifier, emollient, solvent, and humectant.[22] It is a common ingredient in personal care products (eg, cleansers, hair care products, home hair dye kits, deodorants, cosmetics) and is also present in many topical medications to augment penetration of active ingredients.[1,12,22] Another common allergen with emollient properties is lanolin, a wool alcohol derived from sheep fleece used in cosmetics, toiletries, and medicines.[23,24] Lastly, PPD is an allergen most commonly found in permanent hair dyes and semipermanent dyes used for temporary tattoos (eg, black henna).[1,12]

### Allergic Contact Dermatitis Distribution and Associated Allergens

The distribution of ACD can often provide clues regarding the culprit allergen. The initial presentation of ACD is often most informative, because ACD may result in an id reaction, or generalized immune response unassociated with direct skin contact with a culprit allergen, such as with nickel.[25] **Table 2** summarizes common distributions for ACD, frequent causative allergens for each respective distribution, and other common site-specific dermatologic diagnoses to consider in the differential diagnosis.

### Eyelids

The eyelid's thin epidermis makes it prone to ICD and ACD. Common causes of isolated eyelid ACD are shampoos and conditioners, which are rinsed over closed eyelids while showering, then occluded in the eyelid creases when the eyes are open.[3,26,27] Leave-on hair products are more likely to cause dermatitis than rinse-off products.[3] Allergens may be ectopically transferred to the eyelids, such as nail products containing tosylamide formaldehyde resin (nail polishes/hardeners) and acrylates (artificial nails, nail glues). Jewelry comprised of nickel, cobalt, and gold are other common culprits.[26]

Products directly applied to the eyelid can also cause ACD, such as eye shadow or shellac-containing mascara.[3,27] Nickel-plated eyelash curlers and tweezers are sources of metal exposure. Rubber accelerators in the rubber component of eyelash curlers and in foam makeup sponges can also be contributory.[3,26] Additionally, ophthalmic drops contain active (eg, β-blockers) and inactive (eg, preservatives, such as benzalkonium chloride and thimerosal) ingredients that are allergenic. Dermatitis from ophthalmic solutions tends to be more concentrated on the lower eyelid as the product drips down following application.[3,26,28]

Airborne ACD classically presents as eyelid and facial dermatitis with sparing of the nose, which has been referred to as the "beak sign."[29] Products with potential to trigger airborne dermatitis include air fresheners, paints, cleaning products, and insecticides.[1] Plants, such as those within the *Compositae*, or *Asteraceae*, family may also be causative.[1,30,31]

### Scalp/hairline

The scalp is generally resistant to contact dermatitis, and products applied to the scalp often first cause dermatitis of the hairline, eyelids, face, neck, and hands because of ectopic transfer. However, ACD of the scalp is caused by hair dye (PPD), permanent-waving solution (glyceryl thioglycolate), hair clips/clasps (nickel, cobalt), and shampoos/conditioners (preservatives, fragrance, surfactants).[32,33] Adhesives used in wigs, weaves, and extensions can trigger ICD, but rarely ACD. Personal care products applied to the face can cause ACD accentuated at the hairline because of retention of product at the periphery of the face after products are rinsed off.[3]

### Lips/perioral

Contact cheilitis can develop from products directly applied to the lips or to nearby skin or oral mucosa. Erythema that extends beyond the vermillion border is suggestive of contact cheilitis.

Allergy to lip cosmetics (eg, lipstick, lip balm) should be suspected if upper and lower lips are equally and symmetrically affected. Potential allergens include

**Table 2**
**Common allergens and differential diagnosis based on dermatitis distribution**

| Distribution of Dermatitis | Allergens Commonly Associated with ACD in This Distribution | Selected Other Diagnoses to Consider in This Distribution |
|---|---|---|
| Eyelid | Personal care products<br>  Fragrance: fragrance mix I<br>    and II, balsam of Peru, others<br>  Preservatives: MI, MCI/MI,<br>    formaldehyde<br>    and formaldehyde-releasing<br>    preservatives (quaternium-15,<br>    DMDM hydantoin),<br>    iodopropynyl butylcarbamate<br>  Emulsifiers: propylene glycol<br>  Surfactants: cocamidopropyl<br>    betaine,<br>    oleamidopropyl betaine,<br>    amidoamine<br>  Nail products: tosylamide<br>    (toluene) sulfonamide<br>    formaldehyde resin, acrylates<br>Topical antibiotics: neomycin,<br>  bacitracin<br>Metals (eg, jewelry, eyelash<br>  curler): nickel,<br>  cobalt, gold<br>Ophthalmic medications:<br>  β-blockers (eg, timolol),<br>  preservatives (eg, benzalkonium<br>  chloride, thimerosal) | ICD, atopic dermatitis,<br>  seborrheic dermatitis,<br>  psoriasis, rosacea,<br>  dermatomyositis |
| Scalp/hairline | Metals (eg, hair clasps, pins,<br>  brushes):<br>  nickel, cobalt<br>Shampoos and conditioners:<br>  fragrance,<br>  preservatives,<br>Hair dyes: PPD<br>Hair permanent wave solution:<br>  glyceryl thioglycolate | ICD, seborrheic<br>  dermatitis, psoriasis,<br>  atopic dermatitis |
| Lip/perioral | Lip cosmetics: lanolin, propolis,<br>  propyl gallate,<br>  flavoring agents (eg, cinnamic<br>  aldehyde,<br>  carvone, menthol), fragrance,<br>  chemical<br>  sunscreen agents (eg,<br>  oxybenzone)<br>Toothpaste: flavoring agents,<br>  cocamidopropyl<br>  betaine, propylene glycol | ICD (lip licking), atopic<br>  dermatitis, actinic<br>  cheilitis, *Candida* |
| Neck | Personal care products: fragrance,<br>  preservatives,<br>  emulsifiers, surfactants, nail<br>  products (see Eyelid)<br>Topical antibiotics: neomycin,<br>  bacitracin | ICD, atopic dermatitis,<br>  seborrheic dermatitis,<br>  psoriasis |

*(continued on next page)*

**Table 2**
*(continued)*

| Distribution of Dermatitis | Allergens Commonly Associated with ACD in This Distribution | Selected Other Diagnoses to Consider in This Distribution |
|---|---|---|
| | Metals (eg, necklaces, zippers): nickel, cobalt, gold<br>Musical instruments: colophony, propolis, exotic wood<br>Textile: ethylene/melamine formaldehyde resin, disperse blue 106/124 | |
| Axillae | Deodorants and antiperspirants: fragrance, propylene glycol, essential oils, parabens, vitamin E, lanolin – affects axillary vault<br>Metals (eg, released from razors, rare): nickel<br>Textile: ethylene/melamine formaldehyde resin, disperse blue 106/124 – affects axillary rim, sparing the vault | ICD, intertrigo, inverse psoriasis |
| Waistline/ umbilical | Elastic waistbands (eg, clothing, undergarments): rubber accelerators/antioxidants<br>Belts: chromium (leather tanning), p-tert-butylphenol formaldehyde resin (leather and neoprene glue), nickel (belt buckle)<br>Clothing snaps and buttons: nickel | ICD, psoriasis (if umbilical) |
| Shins/calves | Medicaments: topical antibiotics, topical corticosteroids, preservatives, fragrance<br>Bandages and dressings: rubber accelerators, hydrocolloid, topical antibiotics<br>Sports equipment: p-tert-butylphenol formaldehyde resin, acetophenone azine | Stasis dermatitis, ICD |
| Anogenital | Personal care products: fragrance, preservatives, emulsifiers, surfactants (see Eyelid)<br>Medicaments: topical antibiotics, topical anesthetics, corticosteroids<br>Feminine pads: acrylates, colophony<br>Condoms: rubber accelerators | ICD, psoriasis, lichen planus, lichen sclerosus, lichen simplex chronicus |

*(continued on next page)*

| Table 2 (continued) | | |
|---|---|---|
| Distribution of Dermatitis | Allergens Commonly Associated with ACD in This Distribution | Selected Other Diagnoses to Consider in This Distribution |
| Hands | Gloves or rubber products: rubber accelerators/antioxidants (eg, carba mix, thiuram mix, mercaptobenzothiazole, mercapto mix, black rubber mix, mixed dialkyl thioureas) Personal care and cleaning products: fragrance, preservatives, emulsifiers, surfactants (see Eyelid) Metals: nickel, cobalt, gold Topical antibiotics: neomycin, bacitracin Plants: tulipalin in tulips and Peruvian lilies | Atopic dermatitis, dyshidrotic eczema, psoriasis, tinea manuum, dyshidrosiform bullous pemphigoid, pagetoid reticulosis |
| Periungual | Acrylic, shellac nails: acrylates Nail polish/hardeners: tosylamide (toluene) sulfonamide formaldehyde resin, formaldehyde Nail adhesive, dipping powders: cyanoacrylate | ICD, paronychia |
| Feet | Medicaments: topical antibiotics, topical corticosteroids, topical anesthetics, preservatives, fragrance Shoes: leather tanners (eg, chromium, cobalt, formaldehyde), rubber accelerators (eg, carba mix), glues (eg, p-tert-butylphenol formaldehyde resin), metals (eg, nickel, cobalt), dyes (eg, disperse blue 106/124) | ICD, tinea pedis, psoriasis, pagetoid reticulosis |
| Widespread | Plants: urushiol in poison ivy, poison oak, poison sumac Textile: ethylene/melamine formaldehyde resin, disperse blue 106/124 Personal care products (applied broadly): fragrance, preservatives, emulsifiers, surfactants (see Eyelid) | Atopic dermatitis, psoriasis, drug reaction, id (autoeczematization) reaction, eczematous phase bullous pemphigoid, chronic eczematous eruption of the elderly, cutaneous T-cell lymphoma, Sézary syndrome |
| | | (continued on next page) |

**Table 2**
*(continued)*

| Distribution of Dermatitis | Allergens Commonly Associated with ACD in This Distribution | Selected Other Diagnoses to Consider in This Distribution |
|---|---|---|
| Airborne | Plants: Sesquiterpene lactones in Compositae plants (ragweed, sunflowers, chrysanthemums); urushiol in poison ivy, poison oak, poison sumac<br>Dust particles: wood, cement, metals (nickel, silver, mercury, gold, arsenic)<br>Air fresheners: fragrance<br>Paints: acrylates, MCI/MI)<br>Cleaning products: surfactants, fragrance, MI)<br>Insecticides: carba mix, thiuram mix, ethylenediamine dihydrochloride | ICD, seborrheic dermatitis, dermatomyositis, lupus erythematosus, atopic dermatitis |
| Photodistribution | Chemical sunscreen agents: oxybenzone, octocrylene<br>Nonsteroidal anti-inflammatory drugs (applied topically): diclofenac, ketoprofen, etofenamate<br>Antimicrobials: bithionol, chlorhexidine, fenticlor, hexachlorophene | Chronic actinic dermatitis, lupus erythematosus, dermatomyositis, phototoxic drug eruption, polymorphous light eruption, atopic dermatitis |

emollients (eg, lanolin), propolis (beeswax), propyl gallate, flavoring agents (eg, cinnamic aldehyde, carvone, menthol), fragrance, and sunscreen (eg, oxybenzone).[3,34]

Toothpaste-induced ACD typically affects the lower more than the upper lips, and tends to be asymmetric with more extensive involvement at the oral commissure on the side of the dominant hand. Culprit allergens include flavoring agents (eg, carvone, menthol), cocamidopropyl betaine, and propylene glycol.[3,34]

Other notable causes of allergic cheilitis include topical medicaments (eg, antibiotics, corticosteroids) and metals from musical instruments.[3]

*Neck*

The thin epidermis of the neck makes it susceptible to ICD and ACD. Any product that rinses from the face or scalp can result in ACD of the neck, particularly the anterolateral sides because of run-off pattern. Accentuation in the neck folds may be observed because of product accumulation.[3] Allergens in nail products (previously discussed in Eyelids section) can also involve the neck because of direct transfer.

Allergens directly applied to the neck can also result in dermatitis. Fragrance is a common culprit (**Fig. 3**),[35] as is nickel from necklaces and zippers, which may preferentially affect the posterior more than anterior neck.

Dermatitis of the posterior neck can also result from textile allergy, because clothing fits more tightly at the collar.[36] Textile allergies are typically caused by dyes (eg, disperse blue dyes 106/124) and fabric-finishing resins (eg, dimethylol dihydroxyethyleneurea), rather than synthetic or natural fibers.[36] Lastly, violin/viola

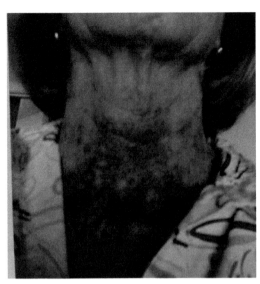

**Fig. 3.** Allergic contact dermatitis to fragrance in perfume can produce the "atomizer sign," a round area of dermatitis overlying the central neck where perfume was sprayed.

players can present with "fiddler's neck," a unilateral neck dermatitis caused by sensitization to the metal brackets attaching the chin rest to the base of the violin/viola, or to materials, such as exotic woods or colophony, used to construct the instrument.[37]

*Axillae*
Chronic occlusion, perspiration, and friction of the axillae may contribute to ICD and ACD. Dermatitis concentrated in the axillary vault should raise consideration for allergy to deodorants and antiperspirants that contain fragrance, propylene glycol, essential oils, parabens, vitamin E, or lanolin.[38] Metals released from razors could trigger dermatitis in the axillary vault, but this is rare because only low amounts of metal are released. Textile allergy (previously discussed in Neck section) should be considered if the dermatitis is primarily located at the anterior or posterior axillary rim where clothing fits more tightly.[3,38]

*Waistline/umbilical*
Waistline ACD is caused by allergens released from articles of clothing and accessories. Rubber accelerators (eg, oxidized chlorine-bleached carbamates) in elastic waistbands can trigger dermatitis, although this is observed less commonly with modern-day clothing and undergarments.[3] Potential allergens from belts include chromium from tanned leather and p-tert-butylphenol formaldehyde resin from glues used to bond leather.[3] Dermatitis localized to the infraumbilical area should raise concern for nickel allergy from belt buckles or clothing fasteners (**Fig. 4**).[3]

*Shins/calves*
Isolated ACD of the shins/calves is most commonly caused by direct application of sensitizing medicaments for stasis dermatitis or leg ulcers. Longer ulcer duration has been associated with increased number of allergen sensitivities.[39] Common sensitizers include preservatives (eg, benzalkonium chloride, propylene glycol, quaternium-15), emollients (eg, lanolin), medicaments (eg, bacitracin, neomycin,

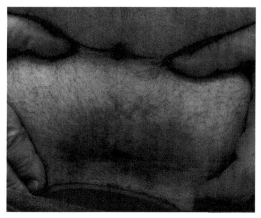

**Fig. 4.** Infraumbilical allergic contact dermatitis from nickel-containing belt buckle.

corticosteroids), and wood tar mix.[3,40] Furthermore, patients can become sensitized to carba mix or other rubber products in bandages and hydrocolloids in wound dressings.

Patients without stasis dermatitis or leg ulcers have been reported to develop ACD to sports equipment, such as shin guards, which may contain allergens, such as p-tert-butylphenol formaldehyde resin.[41] Acetophenone azine is also an increasingly recognized allergen within products made of ethylene vinyl acetate.[42]

*Anogenital*

Anogenital ACD is generally caused by direct application of personal care products, including cleansers, wipes, and lubricants that contain sensitizers, such as preservatives, fragrance, surfactants, and emollients. Topical medicaments that contain anesthetics (eg, benzocaine, dibucaine, lidocaine), antibiotics, and corticosteroids can also be contributory.[43,44] Moreover, spermicides can contain sensitizers, such as hexylresorcinol, nonoxynol-9, oxyquinoline sulfate, phenylmercuric acetate, borate, or quinine hydrochloride.[3] Textile dermatitis can occur in areas where clothing fits tightly. Dietary nickel can also cause anogenital dermatitis (see section on Systemic Contact Dermatitis).

Several allergens can trigger dermatitis of the vulva. For example, feminine pads may contain sensitizing acrylates (used in ultra-absorbent gels), colophony (used to adhere layers of the pad), and rarely, dyes. Ectopic transfer of nail polish or other sensitizers from the hands may also occur. Pessaries, cervical diaphragms, condoms, and other rubber-containing products produce ACD because of sensitivity to antioxidants and accelerators used during manufacturing.

Isolated ACD of the penis is rare, but condoms are contributory. Sensitivity to rubber condoms initially presents as edema of the prepuce, and is triggered by reactions to antioxidants or rubber accelerators used in condom manufacturing. Allergy to vinyl, polyurethane, or lambskin found in nonrubber condoms is rare. Exposure to poison oak or poison ivy often involves the penis; ACD from plants is detailed in the Widespread dermatitis section.[3,44]

*Hands*

Hand dermatitis is common, and one large study showed that more than 30% of patch-tested patients had involvement of the hands.[45] Endogenous factors, such as atopy or decreased skin barrier function, may predispose individuals to developing exogenous hand dermatitis. Contact dermatitis of the hands is more commonly irritant rather than allergic, and wet work has been strongly associated with hand dermatitis.[45] Among those with hand ACD, 40.9% had a concurrent diagnosis of ICD, and 33% had reactions to specifically identifiable relevant irritants, most commonly in the categories of solvents/oils/lubricants/fuels and soaps/cleaners/detergents.[45]

Hand dermatitis is frequently encountered in certain occupational settings. For example, sensitivity to rubber accelerators (eg, thiuram mix, carba mix) associated with glove use is commonly observed in health care workers, operators, mechanics, welders, technicians, and those in the cleaning service.[45] This often presents first with involvement of the dorsal hands and volar wrists. Florists may become sensitized to tulipalin, an allergen found in tulips and Peruvian lilies, which causes fingertip dermatitis of the dominant hand. Furthermore, hairdressers may become sensitized to allergens in hair treatments, such as PPD or glyceryl thioglycolate.[1]

Hand dermatitis is often triggered by a multitude of allergens, such as preservatives, including MI, MCI/MI, quaternium-15, formaldehyde, and iodopropynyl butylcarbamate. Other frequent allergens include nickel, cobalt, gold, fragrance, balsam of Peru, neomycin, and bacitracin. Vesicular hand dermatitis is a manifestation of systemic contact dermatitis (further discussed in the Systemic Contact Dermatitis section).[1,3,45]

### Nails

Rather than involving the nail unit, allergies to nail care products more frequently cause ACD of the face, eyelids, neck, or hands by ectopic transfer.[3] Nail-related dermatitis affects nail technicians and cosmetologists frequently because the allergens not only penetrate gloves, but can also be transferred by airborne exposure.[46]

Historically, the most common allergen in nail polish is tosylamide formaldehyde resin, used to add flexibility and strength and to help polish adhere to the nail.[17] However, prevalence of this allergy has decreased because manufacturers started producing "hypoallergenic" formulations, replacing tosylamide with polyester resins or cellulose acetate butyrate. In addition, the increasing popularity of long-lasting nail polish techniques, such as gel nail polish, containing acrylate allergens may also contribute to this trend.[46] Artificial nails (also referred to as acrylic, gel, solar, or shellac nails) also contain sensitizers, primarily methacrylate monomers, such as methyl methacrylate, ethyl methacrylate, or hydroxyethyl methacrylate. Lastly, adhesives used to attach preformed plastic nails to the nail plate (eg, press-on nails) often contain cyanoacrylate, which is allergenic. Dipping powders also contain cyanoacrylate.[3,46]

### Feet

Foot ACD may occur to medicaments. One common scenario is a patient who develops ICD of the dorsal feet because of excessive friction and sweating, who then self-treats with topical antifungals, antibiotics, and/or corticosteroids that trigger ACD. Dermatitis can persist even after stopping the medicaments, because the creams/ointments remain inside the shoes, resulting in continual contact with the skin.[3]

Besides medicaments, ACD of the feet is caused by allergens used in shoe or stocking manufacturing.[3] Potassium dichromate, a chromium salt used to tan leather, is a frequent shoe-related allergen. Rubber products and dyes, such as PPD, 4-aminoazobenzene, disperse orange 3, and disperse yellow 3, may also be contributory. Adhesive additives, such as p-tert-butylphenol formaldehyde resin and dodecylmercaptan, used to attach shoe linings and insoles, are other common culprits. If the plantar foot is involved, dyes, glues, rubber accelerators (released from insoles), and plastics should be considered.[3,47]

*Widespread*

Plants can trigger a widespread ACD, and the most common culprits are *Toxicodendron* species, which include poison oak, poison ivy, and poison sumac.[48] Urushiol is the allergenic agent. Several distinguishing features can aid in identifying *Toxicodendron* species. First, the leaflets come in triplets (poison oak, poison ivy) or more odd-numbered leaflets (poison sumac). Furthermore, when urushiol oxidizes, it forms polymers that look like "black dots," which are seen on the leaves. Plant-related ACD classically presents with vesicles and bullae arranged in linear streaks caused by the plant brushing against the skin. The allergens often remain on clothing and can result in a widespread dermatitis.[30]

Other causes of generalized ACD include products broadly applied to the skin (eg, soaps, moisturizers) and clothing textiles, which involves such areas as the waistband, medial/lateral thighs, axillary rim, and shoulders.[3] Potassium peroxymonosulfate, a potassium salt found in swimming pool or hot tub disinfectants, has been reported to cause widespread dermatitis sparing areas covered by bathing suits.[49]

### *Systemic Contact Dermatitis*

Systemic contact dermatitis occurs when systemic exposure (eg, orally, intranasally, intravenously) to a cutaneously sensitized allergen triggers a subsequent allergic hypersensitivity reaction.[50] This may present as vesicular hand dermatitis, widespread dermatitis, flare at sites of prior dermatitis, or "baboon syndrome" (erythema and/or dermatitis at the buttocks and intertriginous areas). It can occur especially with systemic ingestion of foods or supplements containing allergens or related substances, with commonly described allergens including nickel, cobalt, chromium, balsam of Peru, propylene glycol, and others. Moreover, medications that individuals become sensitized to via cutaneous exposure (eg, corticosteroids) can result in systemic contact dermatitis after systemic administration.[3] Similarly, cross-reactions can theoretically occur between contact allergens with a para-amino structure (eg, sulfanilamide, PPD, benzocaine) and sulfonamides, resulting in systemic contact dermatitis after systemic exposure to sulfa drugs.[3] Systemic contact dermatitis should be considered when dermatitis persists despite avoidance of cutaneous exposure to identified allergens.

### SUMMARY

Exogenous dermatitis is comprised of ACD and ICD. Rash morphology can help distinguish between environmental and endogenous causes of dermatitis, whereas distribution of the dermatitis can provide clues regarding possible culprit allergens. Patch testing is needed to confirm the diagnosis of ACD, ideally using comprehensive allergen series inclusive of suspected sensitizers.

### CLINICS CARE POINTS

- Exogenous or environmental exposures can cause irritant or ACD, the former being much more common.
- Clinical findings suggestive of exogenous dermatitis include geometric appearance; linearity; asymmetry (although symmetric presentation is also common); and a distribution that is worsening, changing, or atypical for endogenous dermatoses.
- Clinical findings suggestive of ACD include marked itch and spreading of dermatitis beyond the initial area of contact. In contrast, ICD tends to be characterized by burning, stinging, and pain, and may or may not be associated with mild to moderate itch.

- Many common contact allergens, such as preservatives, emollients, dyes, and fragrance, are found in personal care, occupational, and household products. Metals, such as nickel and cobalt, remain common causes of ACD.
- Dermatitis distribution can provide hints regarding potential culprit allergens. It is also important to consider endogenous causes of dermatitis that may have similar patterns.
- Patch testing should be used whenever possible to confirm a diagnosis of ACD, ideally using comprehensive allergen series inclusive of suspected sensitizers. Notably, not all positive patch tests results are relevant, and correlation to the patients' actual exposures is critical. Avoidance of relevant allergens is the mainstay of ACD management.

## DISCLOSURE

The authors have no relevant conflicts of interest to disclose.

## REFERENCES

1. Nixon R, Mowad C, Marks J. Allergic contact dermatitis. In: Bolognia J, Schaffer J, Cerroni L, editors. Dermatology, vol. 1, 4th edition. Elsevier; 2018. p. 242–59.
2. Mowad CM, Anderson B, Scheinman P, et al. Allergic contact dermatitis: patient diagnosis and evaluation. J Am Acad Dermatol 2016;74(6):1029–40.
3. Zirwas M. Clinical aspects of contact dermatitis. In: Fowler J, Zirwas M, editors. Fisher's contact dermatitis. Contact Dermatitis Institute; 2019. p. 45–81.
4. Lim H, Hawk J, Rosen C. Photodermatologic disorders. In: Bolognia J, Schaffer J, Cerroni L, editors. Dermatology, vol. 2, 4th edition. Elsevier; 2018. p. 1548–67.
5. Brasch J, Becker D, Aberer W, et al. Guideline contact dermatitis: S1-Guidelines of the German Contact Allergy Group (DKG) of the German Dermatology Society (DDG), the Information Network of Dermatological Clinics (IVDK), the German Society for Allergology and Clinical Immunology (DGAKI), the Working Group for Occupational and Environmental Dermatology (ABD) of the DDG, the Medical Association of German Allergologists (AeDA), the Professional Association of German Dermatologists (BVDD) and the DDG. Allergo J Int 2014;23(4):126–38.
6. Mowad CM, Anderson B, Scheinman P, et al. Allergic contact dermatitis: patient management and education. J Am Acad Dermatol 2016;74(6):1043–54.
7. Johansen JD, Aalto-Korte K, Agner T, et al. European Society of Contact Dermatitis guideline for diagnostic patch testing: recommendations on best practice. Contact Dermatitis 2015;73(4):195–221.
8. Cohen D. Irritant contact dermatitis. In: Bolognia J, Schaffer J, Cerroni L, editors. Dermatology, vol. 1, 4th edition. Elsevier; 2018. p. 262–72.
9. Kim JJ, Lim HW. Evaluation of the photosensitive patient. Semin Cutan Med Surg 1999;18(4):253–6.
10. DeKoven JG, Warshaw EM, Zug KA, et al. North American Contact Dermatitis Group Patch Test Results: 2015-2016. Dermatitis 2018;29(6):297–309.
11. Larsson-Stymne B, Widstrom L. Ear piercing: a cause of nickel allergy in schoolgirls? Contact Dermatitis 1985;13(5):289–93.
12. T.R.U.E. TEST allergen information. Smart practice dermatology allergy web site 2020. Available at: https://www.smartpractice.com/shop/wa/category?cn=Products-T.R.U.E.-TEST&id=508222&m=SPA. Accessed August 15, 2020.
13. Scheman A, Severson D. American contact dermatitis society contact allergy management program: an epidemiologic tool to quantify ingredient usage. Dermatitis 2016;27(1):11–3.

14. Boyapati A, Tam M, Tate B, et al. Allergic contact dermatitis to methylisothiazolinone: exposure from baby wipes causing hand dermatitis. Australas J Dermatol 2013;54(4):264–7.
15. Johnston GA, Contributing Members of the British Society for Cutaneous A. The rise in prevalence of contact allergy to methylisothiazolinone in the British Isles. Contact Dermatitis 2014;70(4):238–40.
16. Zirwas MJ, Hamann D, Warshaw EM, et al. Epidemic of isothiazolinone allergy in North America: prevalence data from the North American Contact Dermatitis Group, 2013-2014. Dermatitis 2017;28(3):204–9.
17. Voller LM, Persson L, Bruze M, et al. Formaldehyde in "nontoxic" nail polish. Dermatitis 2019;30(4):259–63.
18. Nikle A, Ericson M, Warshaw E. Formaldehyde release from personal care products: chromotropic acid method analysis. Dermatitis 2019;30(1):67–73.
19. Larsen WG. Perfume dermatitis. J Am Acad Dermatol 1985;12(1 Pt 1):1–9.
20. Sasseville D. Neomycin. Dermatitis 2010;21(1):3–7.
21. Sood A, Taylor JS. Bacitracin: allergen of the year. Am J Contact Dermat 2003; 14(1):3–4.
22. McGowan MA, Scheman A, Jacob SE. Propylene glycol in contact dermatitis: a systematic review. Dermatitis 2018;29(1):6–12.
23. Miest RY, Yiannias JA, Chang YH, et al. Diagnosis and prevalence of lanolin allergy. Dermatitis 2013;24(3):119–23.
24. Knijp J, Bruynzeel DP, Rustemeyer T. Diagnosing lanolin contact allergy with lanolin alcohol and Amerchol L101. Contact Dermatitis 2019;80(5):298–303.
25. Silverberg NB, Licht J, Friedler S, et al. Nickel contact hypersensitivity in children. Pediatr Dermatol 2002;19(2):110–3.
26. Rietschel RL, Warshaw EM, Sasseville D, et al. Common contact allergens associated with eyelid dermatitis: data from the North American Contact Dermatitis Group 2003-2004 study period. Dermatitis 2007;18(2):78–81.
27. Zirwas MJ. Contact dermatitis to cosmetics. Clin Rev Allergy Immunol 2019;56(1): 119–28.
28. Grey KR, Warshaw EM. Allergic contact dermatitis to ophthalmic medications: relevant allergens and alternative testing methods. Dermatitis 2016;27(6):333–47.
29. Staser K, Ezra N, Sheehan MP, et al. The beak sign: a clinical clue to airborne contact dermatitis. Dermatitis 2014;25(2):97–8.
30. McGovern T. Dermatoses due to plants. In: Bolognia J, Schaffer J, Cerroni L, editors. Dermatology, vol. 1, 4th edition. Elsevier; 2018. p. 286–303.
31. Schloemer JA, Zirwas MJ, Burkhart CG. Airborne contact dermatitis: common causes in the USA. Int J Dermatol 2015;54(3):271–4.
32. Aleid NM, Fertig R, Maddy A, et al. Common allergens identified based on patch test results in patients with suspected contact dermatitis of the scalp. Skin Appendage Disord 2017;3(1):7–14.
33. Ojo EO, Gowda A, Nedorost S. Scalp dermatitis in patients sensitized to components of hair products. Dermatitis 2019;30(4):264–7.
34. Zug KA, Kornik R, Belsito DV, et al. Patch-testing North American lip dermatitis patients: data from the North American Contact Dermatitis Group, 2001 to 2004. Dermatitis 2008;19(4):202–8.
35. Jacob SE, Castanedo-Tardan MP. A diagnostic pearl in allergic contact dermatitis to fragrances: the atomizer sign. Cutis 2008;82(5):317–8.
36. Ryberg K, Isaksson M, Gruvberger B, et al. Contact allergy to textile dyes in southern Sweden. Contact Dermatitis 2006;54(6):313–21.

37. Myint CW, Rutt AL, Sataloff RT. Fiddler's neck: a review. Ear Nose Throat J 2017; 96(2):76–9.
38. Zirwas MJ, Moennich J. Antiperspirant and deodorant allergy: diagnosis and management. J Clin Aesthet Dermatol 2008;1(3):38–43.
39. Paramsothy Y, Collins M, Smith AG. Contact dermatitis in patients with leg ulcers. The prevalence of late positive reactions and evidence against systemic ampliative allergy. Contact Dermatitis 1988;18(1):30–6.
40. Saap L, Fahim S, Arsenault E, et al. Contact sensitivity in patients with leg ulcerations: a North American study. Arch Dermatol 2004;140(10):1241–6.
41. Herro E, Jacob SE. p-tert-Butylphenol formaldehyde resin and its impact on children. Dermatitis 2012;23(2):86–8.
42. Raison-Peyron N, Bergendorff O, Bourrain JL, et al. Acetophenone azine: a new allergen responsible for severe contact dermatitis from shin pads. Contact Dermatitis 2016;75(2):106–10.
43. Yale K, Awosika O, Rengifo-Pardo M, et al. Genital allergic contact dermatitis. Dermatitis 2018;29(3):112–9.
44. Warshaw EM, Kimyon RS, Silverberg JI, et al. Evaluation of patch test findings in patients with anogenital dermatitis. JAMA Dermatol 2020;156(1):85–91.
45. Warshaw EM, Ahmed RL, Belsito DV, et al. Contact dermatitis of the hands: cross-sectional analyses of North American Contact Dermatitis Group Data, 1994-2004. J Am Acad Dermatol 2007;57(2):301–14.
46. Warshaw EM, Voller LM, Silverberg JI, et al. Contact dermatitis associated with nail care products: retrospective analysis of North American Contact Dermatitis Group Data, 2001-2016. Dermatitis 2020;31(3):191–201.
47. Warshaw EM, Schram SE, Belsito DV, et al. Shoe allergens: retrospective analysis of cross-sectional data from the north american contact dermatitis group, 2001-2004. Dermatitis 2007;18(4):191–202.
48. Kim Y, Flamm A, ElSohly MA, et al. Poison ivy, oak, and sumac dermatitis: what is known and what is new? Dermatitis 2019;30(3):183–90.
49. Kagen MH, Wolf J, Scheman A, et al. Potassium peroxymonosulfate-induced contact dermatitis. Contact Dermatitis 2004;51(2):89–90.
50. Nijhawan RI, Molenda M, Zirwas MJ, et al. Systemic contact dermatitis. Dermatol Clin 2009;27(3):355–64, vii.

# Pediatric Allergic Contact Dermatitis

Christen Brown, BS[a], JiaDe Yu, MD[b,c],*

## KEYWORDS

- Pediatric allergic contact dermatitis • Contact dermatitis • Patch testing
- Pediatric allergy • Allergy • Atopic dermatitis

## KEY POINTS

- Allergic contact dermatitis is equally prevalent in children and in adults, and patch testing is the gold standard for evaluation.
- Children can develop allergic contact dermatitis at any age, even in infancy.
- Children with atopic dermatitis can develop allergic contact dermatitis to weaker allergens found in eczema therapies.
- Patch testing should be performed to a broad baseline series such as the Pediatric Baseline Series in addition to personal products.

## INTRODUCTION

Allergic contact dermatitis (ACD) in children was once thought to be a rare occurrence, but studies have shown that it affects up to 20% of children.[1] Its prevalence and significance within the pediatric population are likely underrepresented because many cases are either undiagnosed or misdiagnosed, unreported, or both.[2,3] ACD may be difficult to distinguish clinically from atopic dermatitis (AD) because of the high prevalence of AD in children. However, in a systematic review and meta-analysis, there was no significant difference in the prevalence of ACD in patients with and without AD.[4,5] Untreated, recalcitrant pediatric ACD can have significant negative consequences on the patients' quality of life, and, thus, expedient referrals for patch testing and adequate clinical suspicion are key to treatment of pediatric ACD. This article presents an update on the most recent literature on pediatric ACD and discusses common contact allergens in children, patch testing techniques, special considerations, and best practices relevant to the point of care.

[a] Tulane University School of Medicine, 1430 Tulane Avenue, New Orleans, LA 70112, USA; [b] Department of Dermatology, Massachusetts General Hospital, Boston, MA, USA; [c] Harvard Medical School, Boston, MA, USA
* Corresponding author. Department of Dermatology, 50 Staniford Street, Suite 200, Boston, MA 02114.
E-mail address: jiade.yu@mgh.harvard.edu
Twitter: @patchtestyu (J.Y.)

Immunol Allergy Clin N Am 41 (2021) 393–408
https://doi.org/10.1016/j.iac.2021.04.004
0889-8561/21/© 2021 Elsevier Inc. All rights reserved.
immunology.theclinics.com

## HISTORY OF PEDIATRIC ALLERGIC CONTACT DERMATITIS

In 1931, Straus[6] first described contact sensitization of infants with an experimental model testing poison ivy in newborns and found that 73% had contact sensitization and developed a delayed type IV hypersensitivity reaction to poison ivy. Subsequent studies investigated the prevalence of positive patch test results in children younger than 5 years of age to determine whether sensitization to contact allergens was as common at a very young age.[3] Bruckner and colleagues[3] used the TRUE (Thin Layer Rapid-Use Epicutaneous, SmartPractice, Phoenix, AZ) test, and found contact sensitization in 24.5% of asymptomatic children, and, pivotally, determined that half of all sensitized children were younger than 18 months of age, reinforcing the idea that sensitization to contact allergens may begin in infancy and is common in older infants and young children.

## EPIDEMIOLOGY OF PEDIATRIC ALLERGIC CONTACT DERMATITIS

The first recent study of pediatric ACD in the United States was published in 2008 from the North American Contact Dermatitis Group (NACDG) based on data collected from 2001 to 2004 in children.[7] They found no significant difference in the overall frequency of positive patch test reactions in children (51.2%) compared with adults (54.1%); however, the allergens differed between the groups, with children more likely to have reactions to nickel, cobalt, thimerosal, and lanolin, whereas adults were more likely to have reactions to neomycin, fragrance mix, balsam of Peru (BoP), and quaternium 15 (a formaldehyde releaser).[7] These differences may be explained by differences in age, and frequency and duration of exposure.[7] Children were also more likely have a comorbid diagnosis of AD than adults.[7]

Since the last NACDG publication in children, the retrospective Pediatric Contact Dermatitis Registry (PCDR) in 2016 reported multicenter data on 1142 children and found that 48% of patients had 1 or more relevant positive patch test.[8] Common allergens included metals (nickel and cobalt), fragrances, antibiotics (including neomycin and bacitracin), propylene glycol, and cocamidopropyl betaine (**Table 1**).[8]

Similar studies have taken place abroad, including the European Surveillance System on Contact Allergies (ESSCA), the largest pediatric ACD study from Europe. The ESSCA collected patch test data from 11 European countries, and 6008 patients aged 1 to 16 years with suspected ACD between 2002 and 2008.[9] There was a 36.9% positive patch test rate.[9] The 10 most frequent allergens are shown in **Table 1**.[9] Younger children aged 1 to 5 years were more likely to be polysensitized compared with older children aged 6 to 16 years.[9] Like other global studies,[10] allergen sensitivities varied by geographic region.[9] There was no difference in prevalence of positive patch test reactions between boys and girls and between children with AD and without.[9]

However, epidemiologic data in children are still incomplete because of underuse of patch testing in children and inconsistent data collection. Work is currently underway at multiple academic centers in the United States to prospectively collect data on pediatric ACD.

## PATHOPHYSIOLOGY OF ALLERGIC CONTACT DERMATITIS

ACD is a cell-mediated inflammatory, biphasic response to cutaneous exposure to allergens.[2,4] During the sensitization phase, the skin is directly exposed to allergens that penetrate the stratum corneum.[2,11] These allergens are subsequently taken up by antigen-presenting cells that migrate to draining lymph nodes, leading to activation of naive T cells that differentiate into primed effector and memory T lymphocytes.[12,13] Although there are no clinical manifestations of the sensitization phase,

**Table 1**
Comparison of Top 10 allergens listed in North American Contact Dermatitis Group, Pediatric Contact Dermatitis Registry, and European Surveillance System on Contact Allergies data

|     | NACDG | PPT (%) | PCDR | PPT (%) | ESSCA | PPT (%) |
| --- | --- | --- | --- | --- | --- | --- |
| 1 | Nickel sulfate | 28.1 | Nickel sulfate | 22.0 | Nickel sulfate | 20.9 |
| 2 | Cobalt dichloride | 12.3 | Fragrance mix I | 11.0 | Cobalt dichloride | 8.3 |
| 3 | Neomycin sulfate | 7.1 | Cobalt dichloride | 9.1 | Potassium dichromate | 5.4 |
| 4 | BoP | 5.7 | BoP | 8.4 | Neomycin sulfate | 4.4 |
| 5 | Lanolin alcohols | 5.5 | Neomycin sulfate | 7.2 | MCI/MI | 3.2 |
| 6 | Fragrance mix I | 5.2 | Propylene glycol | 6.8 | BoP | 3 |
| 7 | Bacitracin | 5.2 | Composite mix | 6.4 | p-Phenylenediamine | 2.5 |
| 8 | Carmine | 3.8 | Bacitracin | 6.2 | Fragrance mix I | 1.9 |
| 9 | p-Phenylenediamine | 3.3 | Formaldehyde | 5.7 | Lanolin alcohols | 1.9 |
| 10 | Quaternium-15 | 3.2 | Gold sodium thiosulfate | 5.7 | Thiuram mix | 1.7 |

*Abbreviations:* BoP, Balsam of Peru; ESSCA, European Surveillance System on Contact Allergies; MCI, methylchloroisothiazolinone; MI, methylisothiazolinone; PPT, positive patch test.

these immune reactions may be ongoing internally for 10 to 15 days.[14,15] The potency of allergens varies, and a single exposure of the more potent allergens (eg, poison ivy) may be sufficient for sensitization to occur.[2,11] Conditions that cause disruption of the skin barrier, such as AD or cutaneous injury, predispose toward sensitization.[2,5,16] The elicitation phase of ACD produces clinical features of the disease. In this phase, reexposure to the sensitized allergen leads to activation and mobilization of primed effector and memory T lymphocytes, producing the localized, erythematous, pruritic, and eczematous eruptions seen in clinical manifestations of ACD.[12,13] Although the pathogenesis of ACD has not been fully elucidated, cytotoxic T, T-helper (Th)1, Th2, Th17, and Th22 cells have all been implicated in the development of ACD.[13,17]

## OVERLAP OF ATOPIC DERMATITIS AND ALLERGIC CONTACT DERMATITIS

AD is the most common chronic inflammatory skin disease in children, affecting up to 13%.[16,18,19] Similar to ACD, the pathogenesis of AD is multifactorial and includes a combination of factors such as genetic predisposition, skin barrier defects, environmental triggers, and an errant immune system.[20,21] AD is primarily mediated by Th2 cells in both the acute and chronic phases, producing pruritic eczematous plaques and patches that make ACD difficult to distinguish from AD.[12,22] The relationship between AD and ACD has not been definitively elucidated. Historically, it was thought that the predominantly Th2 inflammatory response of AD would result in a lower likelihood of ACD, predominantly Th1 mediated.[23] Uehara and Sawai[23] found that contact sensitivity was suppressed in patients with AD who have extensive skin lesions. Earlier studies found that patients with AD who develop ACD require a larger sensitizing dose or repeated applications before showing clinical manifestations.[24] However, some studies have shown that, compared with patients without AD, patients with AD have an increased risk of developing ACD with increased potential to being allergic to multiple, weaker allergens.[21,24,25] This finding is likely caused by the inherent disruption of the skin barrier in AD that leads to increased penetration of irritants and allergens in emollients and topical medication used by patients with AD.[16,26,27] Furthermore, there is also evidence that disruption of the skin barrier (in particular tight junctions) may lead to the expression of danger signals (inflammasomes, toll-like receptors, C-type lecithin receptors, neuropeptide receptors, and so forth) that may lead to cutaneous sensitization to less potent allergens.[28–30]

More recently, in a retrospective case review of 1142 children, patients with AD were more likely to react to allergens found in their skin care products (eg, cocamidopropyl betaine, wool alcohol [lanolin], tixocortol-21-pivalate, and Compositae-related allergens).[25] These data are significant in that they present a challenge to clinicians who must consider the possibility of superimposed ACD in patients with AD. The study also showed that children who presented for patch testing, and who also had an underlying history of AD, tended to be (1) younger than their counterparts without AD, (2) more likely to present with generalized dermatitis, (3) have prolonged duration of dermatitis compared with those without, and (4) that Asians and African Americans with ACD were also more likely to have concurrent AD.[25] Thus, although the nature of the relationship between ACD and AD continues to be debated, there are increasing data in the literature that show that ACD can coincide with and exacerbate the clinical course of AD

## PHYSICAL EXAMINATION CLUES TO ALLERGIC CONTACT DERMATITIS IN CHILDREN

Given the high prevalence of AD in children and the overlapping clinical features of ACD and AD, differentiating between them can be a challenge. There are key clinical findings that may suggest ACD: if a patient's dermatitis (1) worsens despite usual treatment and/or changes distribution; (2) becomes recalcitrant to current treatments; (3) presents in unusual locations, such as predominantly the head and neck, hand or foot, eyelid, groin, perioral, or periorbital; (4) commences in adolescence with no history of childhood eczema; (5) requires immunosuppressive systemic medication; and (6) rebounds after cessation of therapy.[16,31] In some circumstances, patients can be sensitized to the active ingredients in their topical therapies, leading to rebound of their dermatitis.[16,31] A helpful algorithm for patch testing in children has been published that may be used to guide clinical decision making.[12]

The location of rash and clinical history may provide clues to specific allergens. According to the NACDG, the most common sites for pediatric ACD are the face, generalized scattered distribution pattern, and extremities (arms and legs).[32] Facial dermatitis in children may be caused by common personal care products such as shampoos, soaps, and face creams, which may contain preservatives, fragrances, and surfactants.[33,34] Often, more than 1 allergen can contribute to dermatitis in the same distribution (eyelids, periorbital), such as benzoyl peroxide in acne wash and diethylthiourea, the rubber accelerator found in equipment (goggles, masks, wetsuits) used in water sports.[35] Hand dermatitis in children may be associated with various sources, ranging from a popular homemade toy called slime, which is made with common household products, including glues, detergents, and soaps, to personal care products such as moisturizers, hand soap, and nail polish.[33,36] Dermatitis of the extremities may be a result of shin guards used in contact sports, which contain allergens such as neoprene rubbers or glues.[12,33] Dermatitis affecting diaper areas is another method to differentiate ACD from AD in children, because this region is usually spared in AD.[11,37] Face dermatitis could result from electronic devices that contain nickel, cosmetics, spray-on fragrances, or common personal care items such as face washes and moisturizers.[33,37]

## PATCH TESTING SERIES FOR CHILDREN

Patch testing is the gold standard for diagnosis of ACD, but, despite the increasing prevalence of children with ACD, testing is less used in children. The PCDR showed that, although patch test evaluations occur in children as young as 7 months, and that most providers customize their patch tests to patient history, most providers patch tested fewer than 10 patients annually.[8] In the most recent study by the NACDG in adults from 2015 to 2016, more than 5597 adults were tested.[38] However, over 8 years, only 883 children were tested by the NACDG, a difference of nearly 25-fold.[38] The discrepancy in patch testing between adults and children may be caused by barriers that limit patch testing capabilities in the pediatric population, including lack of consensus on allergens to patch test in children, misdiagnosis of ACD, logistical challenges, and general knowledge gap on how to patch test in children.

In 2017, The TRUE test was approved by the US Food and Drug Administration in children aged 6 to 18 years.[38,39] The TRUE test is a commercially available patch test kit containing 35 allergens, and 1 study found that it detects only 67% of the most common allergens.[38] Some prevalent allergens in children, such as methylisothiazolinone (MI), propylene glycol, and cocamidopropyl betaine, are not included in the TRUE test. Clinicians also are unable to add or subtract allergens from the TRUE test, making customization based on patient history impossible. Although the TRUE test is a reasonable screening test for patients suspected of having ACD, more comprehensive testing is necessary to avoid missing relevant allergens.

To facilitate comprehensive patch testing in children, an expert consensus-derived baseline patch test series for children aged 6 to 18 years was published in 2017.[39] The panel includes 38 allergens prevalent in children older than 6 years, and integrates data published by the PCDR and NACDG.[8,32,39] The Pediatric Baseline Series includes high-yield allergens in children in patches that could easily fit on the back of a 6-year-old.[39] Furthermore, the Pediatric Baseline Series is constantly reevaluated in order to add and remove allergens based on changing prevalence data.[39] Ultimately, baseline series such as this serve as a foundation for increasing the diagnostic yield of patch testing in children and detecting emerging allergens in children.

Regionally specific pediatric series are also used in both Australia and Europe. The Australian Pediatric Baseline panel includes 30 allergens based on local prevalence data.[40] The European Academy of Allergy and Clinical Immunology proposed a patch test series in children that included only 9 allergens, with an optional 12 additional allergens available to be used according to history and exposure.[41] Because exposure and allergen prevalence differ between the United States, Australia, and Europe, use of regional baseline series is generally recommended.

## PATCH TESTING PROCEDURE

The process of patch testing in children requires cutaneous application of allergens on the patient's back and avoiding the spine because of movement.[33,37] In addition to the back, patches can be placed on the thighs if the back is not clear for patch testing or if additional space is needed.[37] Although the number of allergens that can be tested is limited by the child's size, it has been estimated that 80 allergens can comfortably fit on an average 8-year-old[37] (**Fig. 1**). Hypoallergenic adhesive tape, such as Scanpor (SmartPractice, Phoenix, AZ) is applied over the patches to avoid dislodging.[37] In smaller children, the number of patches used should be judiciously selected and based on exposure history.[33,34,37] Because younger children may be more susceptible to irritant reactions, shorter occlusion time, such as 24 hours instead of the standard 48 hours, has been proposed, although clinical studies have yet to determine whether

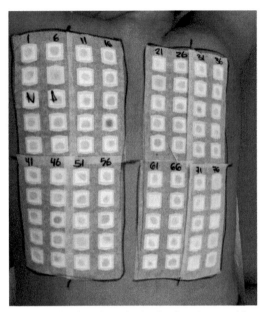

**Fig. 1.** Eighty patches are easily placed on the back of an 8-year-old.

this significantly affects outcomes. Children 13 years of age or older may be patch tested under the same guidelines as adults, with removal of patches and an initial reading at 48 hours, and a second or final reading at 96 hours.[33,37] This final reading is the most clinically relevant reading, with one-third of negative allergen tests at the initial 48-hour reading becoming positive at 96 hours.[33,42] Final reading times may vary from 72 hours to 120 hours, and there is currently no evidence to suggest which time frame is superior, and all may be acceptable. The International Contact Dermatitis Research Group established a standardized grading system for evaluation of patch tests that is widely used.[33,42,43] This grading system entails 6 reaction categories: negative reaction (−); doubtful reaction characterized by faint erythema only (+/−); weak positive reaction with nonvesicular erythema, infiltration, and possible papules (+); strong positive reaction with vesicular erythema, infiltration, and papules (++); and extreme positive reaction with intense erythema and infiltration, coalescing vesicles, and bullous reaction (+++).[33]

Optimal reading times depend on specific allergens. Metals (nickel, cobalt, gold, chromate, palladium), medications (neomycin, topical corticosteroids, caine mix), and certain preservatives and glues (methylchloroisothiazolinone [MCI]/MI, epoxy resin) can be associated with late reactions[33,44] and should be considered for delayed reading at 7 to 10 days after patch test application.[45,46] In comparison, some allergens may have early positive reaction readings that disappear at later readings. Fragrances and preservatives are prominent on day 5 but may disappear by day 7.[33,42]

False-positive and false-negative reactions can occur, and there are many variables that contribute to the strength and clinical relevance of reactions. False-positive reactions are produced when allergens are applied at high irritant concentrations or when patch testing occurs on skin with active dermatitis.[33,34] A phenomenon called angry-back syndrome occurs when false-positive reactions occur adjacent to large true-positive reactions, inducing adjacent skin inflammation and irritation.[34,47] In the setting of angry-back reactions, it is recommended that patch testing be repeated avoiding the strong positive reactions. Importantly, a positive reaction does not always signify a relevant reaction because a positive reaction may have no bearing on the current dermatitis but may be of past relevance. It is important that clinicians incorporate patient history and knowledge of the allergen's likely sources when making an assessment of clinical relevance.[48] Clinical relevance based on positive patch tests depend on current or past exposures,[33,34] and there are 3 categories of relevance. Clinical relevance is definite if the patch test or use test with the offending product is positive.[33,34,42] Clinical relevance is probable if the patch test is positive, the offending allergen is present in known cutaneous exposures, and the clinical presentation aligns with that exposure.[33,34] Clinical relevance is possible if the patch test is positive and the patient has been in contact with materials that may have contained the allergen.[34,44] False-negative reactions may occur when inadequate allergen concentrations are used, when patients are concurrently on immunosuppressive therapy, or when patients have recently been exposed to ultraviolet light in the setting of sun tanning or phototherapy.[33]

### Top 10 Allergens in Children

The top 10 allergens from the PCDR among pediatric patients with suspected ACD are listed in **Table 2**.[8] One European study assessed the prevalence of allergens in supposedly hypoallergenic/tested/safe cosmetics designed for children younger than 1 year and found that 85% contained potential allergens.[49]

Nickel is a ubiquitous metal and is the most common cause of pediatric ACD worldwide.[50,51] One study estimated that 1.1 million children are sensitized to nickel, but this

**Table 2**
**Top 10 allergens by positive patch test and associated sources**

| Allergen Type | Allergen | Sources |
| --- | --- | --- |
| Metal | Nickel sulfate | Jewelry, toys, clothes, belt buckles, electronics |
| | Cobalt dichloride | Pigmented cosmetics, jewelry, dental casting alloys |
| | Gold sodium thiosulfate | Jewelry, dental implants |
| Fragrances | Fragrance mix I | Cosmetics, personal hygiene products |
| | Myroxylon pereirae (BoP) | |
| Preservatives | Formaldehyde and releasers <br> • Quaternium-15 <br> • Diazolidinyl urea <br> • DMDM hydantoin <br> • Imidazolidinyl urea <br> • Bronopol | Personal hygiene products, cleaning supplies |
| | MI and MCI | Household cleaners, hair conditioners, fabric softeners |
| Emollients | Wool (wax) alcohols/lanolin | Emollients, baby and bath oils, hand sanitizers |
| Topical medication | Neomycin sulfate Bacitracin | Topical antibiotics |

Abbreviation: DMDM, 1,3-dimethylol-5, 5-dimethyl hydantoin.

may be an underestimation.[51] Because nickel is common in children's items such as earrings, toys, clothes, belts, and electronics, early exposure to the metal creates opportunity for lifelong sensitization.[52,53] Pediatric-specific data from the NACDG showed that 23.7% of children had positive patch testing to nickel between 1994 and 2014.[50] Girls were significantly more likely to have nickel allergy compared with boys, and jewelry was deemed the most common exposure associated with nickel allergy. Notably, the temporal and environmental contexts of nickel exposure may have some influence on sensitization. One study showed that less sensitization to nickel occurred if metal dental braces were placed before ear piercing.[52] Avoidance strategies include education that enables patients to recognize materials high in nickel content, and wearing jewelry alternatives, including sterling silver, pure yellow gold, platinum, or plastic earrings (alternatives that have little to no nickel content).[53] Patients can also check whether an object releases nickel by using the dimethylglyoxime test kits. If an object releases nickel, the test solution turns pink. Cobalt is found in blue-pigmented cosmetics, jewelry, and dental casting alloys.[37] Cobalt is often found with nickel and therefore cosensitization is common. Gold is found in jewelry and some dental implants.[54]

Fragrance allergens (fragrance mix 1, BoP) are commonly found in cosmetics and personal hygiene products. Israeli researchers found increasing rates of fragrance allergy in children, which they attributed to children using a wider range of cosmetics earlier in life.[55] Younger children who may not yet apply cosmetic products to their own skins may be prone to contact allergy and react to fragrances by proxy of transmission from adults.[55] Misleading marketing terms that present products as being natural or unscented may contain fragrances and contribute to increasing rates of contact sensitization in young children.

Neomycin is a common topical antibiotic used to treat cutaneous infections and sold over the counter in the United States. It is also used as eye and ear drops in children.[2,56] It is frequently used with bacitracin, which is therefore a cosensitizer with neomycin, having similar rates of positive patch test reaction.

Lanolin (wood alcohols) is an allergen found in emollients, baby and bath oil, hand sanitizers, and creams.[57] It is derived from sheep wool,[58,59] and it is a mixture of sterols, fatty alcohols, and fatty acids with varied composition.[60] Given its emollient properties and its prevalence in common hygiene products, ACD can develop after repeated exposure and is particularly common in damaged skin affected by AD.[26,60] Although lanolin alcohol 30% petrolatum is the standard patch test agent used in diagnosing lanolin contact allergy, some studies have shown that additional patch testing with lanolin derivatives may enhance identification of patients with lanolin contact allergy.[58,61,62] One derivative of note, Amerchol L101 50% pet., is a mixture of mineral oil and 10% lanolin alcohols.[63,64] Studies have found more positive reactions to Amerchol L101 than to lanolin alcohol alone.[58,61,64,65] Testing to Amerchol L101 is recommended in pediatric patients.

Formaldehyde and MI are preservatives commonly used to prolong the shelf-life of cosmetic and household products and prevent bacterial, fungal, and viral growth.[37] MI was introduced into the United States market in the 1980s in a 3:1 MCI/MI formulation, but this formulation was gradually replaced by MI alone because of concerns for contact allergy from MCI.[66,67] Thus, high concentrations of MI in particular have become ubiquitous in consumer products over the past decade and can be found in various personal care products, including shampoos, hair conditioners, moisturizers, soaps, and nail polish.[36,68,69] It is also found in household products, including laundry detergents and fabric softeners, and surface disinfectants as well as residential wall paints and glues.[70–73] The American Contact Dermatitis Society (ACDS) named MI the contact allergen of the year in 2013 because of rapidly increasing prevalence.[67] After nickel, it is now the second most common cause of ACD in adults and children.[37] In the United States and Europe, it has replaced potentially carcinogenic preservatives such as formaldehyde.[66] Thus, although MI is known to be a sensitizer and common cause of ACD in adults, cases of pediatric ACD caused by MI are increasing because of its common use in care products for babies and children.[66] MI was found in wet wipes but has been removed because of published cases.[74–76] Recently, an epidemic of hand rash was caused by children making slime using laundry detergent, glues, and soap, all of which may contain MI.[37,73,77,78] MI sensitization is often underdiagnosed in the United States because it is still tested in combination with MCI when using the TRUE test, suggesting a need for MI to be tested singly to prevent missing this important allergen.[66]

Formaldehyde is one of the oldest and most widely used preservatives. It is a ubiquitous allergen that is difficult to avoid given its common placement in many consumer products, including cosmetic, household, and industrial products.[79–81] Thus, it was named as the ACDS Allergen of the Year in 2015.[82] In addition to formaldehyde, preservatives that release formaldehyde, such as quaternium-15, imidazolidinyl urea, diazolidinyl urea, bronopol, and 1,3-dimethylol-5, 5-dimethyl hydantoin (DMDM) hydantoin, are frequently found in personal care products.[79,82,83] One study found that these releasers are among the most frequent allergens in children who underwent patch testing because of ACD, further highlighting the necessity of paying attention to all preservatives included within cosmetic, household, and industrial products on labels.[84]

### Emerging Allergens

New potential allergens are constantly being introduced to consumers, whereas older known allergens are used less frequently, such as MCI. Therefore, it is important to keep track of and test for emerging allergens in children.

Hydroperoxides of limonene and hydroperoxides of linalool are two emerging pediatric fragrance allergens that were found to be positive in 13% and 17.9% of children, respectively, in 1 study.[85] Limonene and linalool are naturally occurring fragrances that rapidly oxidize into their respective hydroperoxides, which are more allergenic than the reduced forms.[85] It is estimated that 60% to 70% of sensitizations to linalool and 70% of sensitizations to limonene were not detected by positive patch test reactions when tested for fragrance allergy alone (fragrance mixes I and II, BoP).[86,87] These fragrances are commonly used in soaps, shampoos, perfumes, and household cleaning products.[86] Limonene has been identified in 88 of 91 essential oils that have caused ACD, and linalool has been identified in 82 of 91 essential oils that have caused ACD.[86,87]

Isobornyl acrylate, an acrylate derivative found in glucose sensors or insulin sets used in the management of type 1 diabetes, is another emerging allergen that should be considered in children.[88] Although medical devices have significantly improved glycemic control and quality of life, cases of adhesive-driven ACD have been reported in association with certain brands of continuous glucose monitors.[89–92] It is thought that isobornyl acrylate leaches through the adhesives to cause sensitization,[93] and this process may be exacerbated by occlusion and sweating.[88] Therefore, it is recommended that isobornyl acrylate should be tested in every suspected case of ACD caused by medical device adhesives or glues to avoid missing sources of sensitization.[88] These findings also highlight the need for increased transparency from manufacturers regarding the agents used to create these medical devices. Isobornyl acrylate was named ACDS Contact Allergen of the Year in 2020.[94]

Acetophenone azine, a biocide found in foam, including sneakers and shin pads, has emerged as a source of ACD presenting in the distribution of the shin and foot, especially in athletes.[95,96] Recently, Darrigade and colleagues[95] reported on 6 male children, aged 7 to 14 years, who presented with shin and plantar dermatitis related to wearing shin pads that contained acetophenone azine. Avoidance strategies for acetophenone azine include wearing leather-inlay soles and using polyurethane shin pads.[95] Of note, many of the children reported in this study had been misdiagnosed as experiencing exacerbation of AD or experiencing recalcitrant hyperkeratotic plantar foot dermatitis.[95] Therefore, it is important to consider patch testing acetophenone azine in children presenting with shin and/or foot dermatitis.[97] Acetophenone azine is an important emerging allergen and will be the ACDS Contact Allergen of the Year in 2021.[98]

### Counseling, Education, Avoidance

Accurate diagnosis with patch testing, avoidance of potential allergens, and future preventive measures are the 3 pillars of pediatric ACD management and treatment.[25,37] Providers should counsel on avoidance and prevention strategies with both the patient and all relevant caretakers,[37] along with initiating treatments that will suppress inflammation (with topical corticosteroids, compresses, topical immunomodulators).[99] National organizations have provided resources to aid with patient counseling. The ACDS offers services to help providers and patients identify common sources of allergens.[14] One such service, the Contact Allergen Management Program (CAMP), is a Web-based resource that assists patients in the management of ACD and aids in identifying which personal care products are safe to use.[100] After patch testing identifies allergens the patient may react to, physicians can generate a personalized list of products that are free of the identified allergens.[100] The patient is also provided with allergen search codes that are tied to the patient's specific allergy profile.[100] Each allergen is linked to synonyms and cross-reactors, and this resource is designed to populate safe alternatives to each allergen.[101]

It must be noted that patch testing is not possible in all patients because of barriers to access and availability of patch testing.[8] Patch testing can also be complicated by having a full-body rash leading to no clear skin for placement of patches, angry-back reaction during patch testing, and false-negatives caused by the use of systemic immunosuppressants at the time of patch testing. Hill and colleagues[102] proposed the option of using a preemptive avoidance strategy (PEAS) in patients who do not have access to patch testing or are highly reactive to patch tests. PEAS is defined as preemptively avoiding the top offending allergens in pediatric ACD in the absence of patch testing.[99,102] The top 10 allergens identified in PEAS were fragrance mix I, BoP, neomycin sulfate, bacitracin, lanolin, formaldehyde, MI, bronopol, propylene glycol, and MCI/MI.[103] The study consisted of a systematic review of 5 studies reporting data on rates of positive patch tests in pediatric patients and estimated that between one-quarter and one-third of these patients theoretically would have had their relevant allergens avoided had they applied the PEAS in careful selection of pediatric personal care products.[102] It is thought that using PEAS for children without access to patch testing may provide an early opportunity for intervention in ACD.[102] Recently, Brankov and colleagues[103] performed a meta-analysis of the most recent data released by the NACDG and PCDR to create a list of the top 25 allergens with high clinical relevance to be considered when using PEAS. New to the list were glucosides, which are found in several products ranging from shampoo to sunscreen, and are marketed at children.[103]

### SUMMARY

ACD can be a physically, psychologically, and economically burdensome disease that has ramifications for both pediatric patients and their caregivers. Children can become sensitized to allergens at an early age, and it is important to have high clinical suspicion of ACD in children of all ages who have recalcitrant dermatitis despite appropriate treatment or who present with dermatitis in an atypical distribution. Accurate and early diagnosis, avoidance, and prevention are key to successful management and treatment of pediatric ACD. There is currently a multicenter North American prospective pediatric ACD registry to gather cases of pediatric ACD from major academic centers across the United States, Canada, and Mexico. Initiatives such as this contribute to elucidating the true prevalence of ACD in children as well as identifying ever-changing trends of allergen sensitization in children. Continued collection of prevalence data is necessary to help guide physician decision making, patient education, and potential industry and governmental response to emerging and evolving contact allergens in children.

## CLINICS CARE POINTS

- Allergic contact dermatitis is prevalent in children and those with atopic dermatitis.
- Patch testing with too limited a series may miss important allergens.
- Patch testing in young children (< 8 years old) require shorter contact time due to risk of irritation.

## DISCLOSURE

The authors report no relevant financial or commercial conflicts with this article.

## REFERENCES

1. Weston WL, Weston JA, Kinoshita J, et al. Prevalence of positive epicutaneous tests among infants, children, and adolescents. Pediatrics 1986;78(6):1070–4.
2. Militello G, Jacob SE, Crawford GH. Allergic contact dermatitis in children. Curr Opin Pediatr 2006;18(4):385–90.
3. Bruckner AL, Weston WL, Morelli JG. Does sensitization to contact allergens begin in infancy? Pediatrics 2000;105(1):e3.
4. Schena D, Papagrigoraki A, Tessari G, et al. Allergic contact dermatitis in children with and without atopic dermatitis. Dermatitis 2012;23(6):275–80.
5. Hamann CR, Hamann D, Egeberg A, et al. Association between atopic dermatitis and contact sensitization: a systematic review and meta-analysis. J Am Acad Dermatol 2017;77(1):70–8.
6. Straus HW. Artificial sensitization of infants to poison ivy. J Allergy 1931;2(3): 137–44.
7. Zug KA, McGinley-Smith D, Warshaw EM, et al. Contact allergy in children referred for patch testing: North American contact dermatitis group data, 2001-2004. Arch Dermatol 2008;144(10):1329–36.
8. Goldenberg A, Mousdicas N, Silverberg N, et al. Pediatric contact dermatitis registry inaugural case data. Dermatitis 2016;27(5):293–302.
9. Belloni Fortina A, Cooper SM, Spiewak R, et al. Patch test results in children and adolescents across Europe. Analysis of the ESSCA Network 2002-2010. Pediatr Allergy Immunol 2015;26(5):446–55.
10. Boonchai W, Chaiyabutr C, Charoenpipatsin N, et al. Pediatric contact allergy: a comparative study with adults. Contact Dermatitis 2021;84(1):34–40.

11. Milingou M, Tagka A, Armenaka M, et al. Patch tests in children: a review of 13 years of experience in comparison with previous data. Pediatr Dermatol 2010; 27(3):255–9.

12. Tam I, Yu J De. Allergic contact dermatitis in children: recommendations for patch testing. Curr Allergy Asthma Rep 2020;20(9):41.

13. Rustemeyer T, Van Hoogstraten IMW, Von Blomberg BME, et al. Mechanisms of irritant and allergic contact dermatitis. In: Johansen JD, Frosch PJ, Lepoittevin J, editors. Contact dermatitis. 5th edition. London and New York: Springer Berlin Heidelberg; 2011. p. 43–90.

14. Goldenberg A, Silverberg N, Silverberg JI, et al. Pediatric allergic contact dermatitis: lessons for better care. J Allergy Clin Immunol Pract 2015;3(5): 661–8.

15. Saint-Mezard P, Rosieres A, Krasteva M, et al. Allergic contact dermatitis. Eur J Dermatol 2004;14(5):284–95.

16. Owen JL, Vakharia PP, Silverberg JI. The role and diagnosis of allergic contact dermatitis in patients with atopic dermatitis. Am J Clin Dermatol 2018;19(3): 293–302.

17. Eyerich K, Eyerich S. Th22 cells in allergic disease. Allergo J Int 2015;24(1):1–7.

18. Odhiambo JA, Williams HC, Clayton TO, et al. Global variations in prevalence of eczema symptoms in children from ISAAC Phase Three. J Allergy Clin Immunol 2009;124(6):1251–8.e23.

19. Garg N, Silverberg JI. Epidemiology of childhood atopic dermatitis. Clin Dermatol 2015;33(3):281–8.

20. Kim J, Kim BE, Leung DYM. Pathophysiology of atopic dermatitis: clinical implications. Allergy Asthma Proc 2019;40(2):84–92.

21. Herro EM, Matiz C, Sullivan K, et al. Frequency of contact allergens in pediatric patients with atopic dermatitis. J Clin Aesthet Dermatol 2011;4(11):39–41.

22. Puar N, Chovatiya R, Paller AS. New treatments in atopic dermatitis. Ann Allergy Asthma Immunol 2020;126(1):21–3.

23. Uehara M, Sawai T. A longitudinal study of contact sensitivity in patients with atopic dermatitis. Arch Dermatol 1989;125(3):366–8.

24. Jones HE, Lewis CW, Mcmarlin SL. Allergic contact sensitivity in atopic dermatitis. Arch Dermatol 1973;107(2):217–22.

25. Jacob SE, McGowan M, Silverberg NB, et al. Pediatric contact dermatitis registry data on contact allergy in children with atopic dermatitis. JAMA Dermatol 2017;153(8):765–70.

26. Thyssen JP, McFadden JP, Kimber I. The multiple factors affecting the association between atopic dermatitis and contact sensitization. Allergy Eur J Allergy Clin Immunol 2014;69(1):28–36.

27. Kohli N, Nedorost S. Inflamed skin predisposes to sensitization to less potent allergens. J Am Acad Dermatol 2016;75(2):312–7.e1.

28. Kuo IH, Yoshida T, De Benedetto A, et al. The cutaneous innate immune response in patients with atopic dermatitis. J Allergy Clin Immunol 2013; 131(2):266–78.

29. Brandner JM, Zorn-Kruppa M, Yoshida T, et al. Epidermal tight junctions in health and disease. Tissue Barriers 2015;3(1):e974451.

30. Ainscough JS, Frank Gerberick G, Dearman RJ, et al. Danger, intracellular signaling, and the orchestration of dendritic cell function in skin sensitization. J Immunotoxicol 2013;10(3):223–34.

31. Chen JK, Jacob SE, Nedorost ST, et al. A pragmatic approach to patch testing atopic dermatitis patients: clinical recommendations based on expert consensus opinion. Dermatitis 2016;27(4):186–92.

32. Zug KA, Pham AK, Belsito DV, et al. Patch testing in children from 2005 to 2012: results from the North American contact dermatitis group. Dermatitis 2014; 25(6):345–55.

33. Schmidlin K, Sani S, Bernstein DI, et al. Clinical management review a hands-on approach to contact dermatitis and patch testing. J Allergy Clin Immunol Pract 2020;8(6):1883–93.

34. Fonacier L. A practical guide to patch testing. J Allergy Clin Immunol Pract 2015;3(5):669–75.

35. Brooks CD, Kujawska A, Patel D. Cutaneous allergic reactions induced by sporting activities. Sport Med 2003;33(9):699–708.

36. Kullberg SA, Gupta R, Warshaw EM. Methylisothiazolinone in children's nail polish. Pediatr Dermatol 2020;37(4):745–7.

37. Tam I, Yu J De. Pediatric contact dermatitis: what's new. Curr Opin Pediatr 2020; 32(4):524–30.

38. DeKoven JG, Warshaw EM, Zug KA, et al. North American contact dermatitis group patch test results: 2015-2016. Dermatitis 2018;29(6):297–309.

39. Yu J, Atwater AR, Brod B, et al. Pediatric baseline patch test series: pediatric contact dermatitis workgroup. Dermatitis 2018;29(4):206–12.

40. Felmingham C, Davenport R, Bala H, et al. Allergic contact dermatitis in children and proposal for an Australian Paediatric baseline series. Australas J Dermatol 2020;61(1):33–8.

41. de Waard-van der Spek FB, Darsow U, Mortz CG, et al. EAACI position paper for practical patch testing in allergic contact dermatitis in children. Pediatr Allergy Immunol 2015;26(7):598–606.

42. Fonacier L, Bernstein DI, Pacheco K, et al. Contact dermatitis: a practice parameter-update 2015. J Allergy Clin Immunol Pract 2015;3(3 Suppl):S1–39.

43. Wilkinson DS, Fregert S, Magnusson B, et al. Terminology of contact dermatitis. Acta Derm Venereol 1970;50(4):287–92.

44. Fonacier L, Noor I. Contact dermatitis and patch testing for the allergist. Ann Allergy Asthma Immunol 2018;120(6):592–8.

45. Matiz C, Russell K, Jacob SE. The importance of checking for delayed reactions in pediatric patch testing. Pediatr Dermatol 2011;28(1):12–4.

46. Dickel H, Taylor JS, Evey P, et al. Delayed readings of a standard screening patch test tray: Frequency of "lost," "found," and "persistent" reactions. Am J Contact Dermat 2000;11(4):213–7.

47. Duarte I, Lazzarini R, Bedrikow R. Excited skin syndrome: Study of 39 patients. Am J Contact Dermat 2002;13(2):59–65.

48. Bourke J, Coulson I, English J. Guidelines for the management of contact dermatitis: An update. Br J Dermatol 2009;160(5):946–54.

49. Dumycz K, Kunkiel K, Feleszko W. Cosmetics for neonates and infants: Haptens in products' composition. Clin Transl Allergy 2019;9:15.

50. Warshaw EM, Aschenbeck KA, DeKoven JG, et al. Epidemiology of pediatric nickel sensitivity: Retrospective review of North American Contact Dermatitis Group (NACDG) data 1994-2014. J Am Acad Dermatol 2018;79(4):664–71.

51. Rietschel RL, Fowler JF, Warshaw EM, et al. Detection of nickel sensitivity has increased in North American patch-test patients. Dermatitis 2008;19(1):16–9.

52. Mortz CG, Lauritsen JM, Bindslev-Jensen C, et al. Nickel sensitization in adolescents and association with ear piercing, use of dental braces and hand eczema:

The odense adolescence cohort study on atopic diseases and dermatitis (TOACS). Acta Derm Venereol 2002;82(5):359–64.

53. Silverberg NB, Pelletier JL, Jacob SE, et al. Nickel allergic contact dermatitis: Identification, treatment, and prevention. Pediatrics 2020;145(5).

54. Silverberg NB. The "jewelry Addict": allergic contact dermatitis from repetitive multiple children's jewelry exposures. Pediatr Dermatol 2016;33(2):e103–5.

55. Zafrir Y, Trattner A, Hodak E, et al. Patch testing in Israeli children with suspected allergic contact dermatitis: a retrospective study and literature review. Pediatr Dermatol 2018;35(1):76–86.

56. Seidenari S, Giusti F, Pepe P, et al. Contact sensitization in 1094 children undergoing patch testing over a 7-year period. Pediatr Dermatol 2005;22(1):1–5.

57. Admani S, Jacob SE. Allergic contact dermatitis in children: Review of the past decade. Curr Allergy Asthma Rep 2014;14(4):421.

58. Lee B, Warshaw E. Lanolin allergy: history, epidemiology, responsible allergens, and management. Dermatitis 2008;19(2):63–72.

59. Schlossman ML, McCarthy JP. Lanolin and derivatives chemistry: relationship to allergic contact dermatitis. Contact Dermatitis 1979;5(2):65–72.

60. Knijp J, Bruynzeel DP, Rustemeyer T. Diagnosing lanolin contact allergy with lanolin alcohol and Amerchol L101. Contact Dermatitis 2019;80(5). cod.13210.

61. Miest RYN, Yiannias JA, Chang Y-HH, et al. Diagnosis and prevalence of lanolin allergy. Dermatitis 2013;24(3):119–23.

62. Mortensen T. Allergy to lanolin. Contact Dermatitis 1979;5(3):137–9.

63. Fransen M, Overgaard LEK, Johansen JD, et al. Contact allergy to lanolin: temporal changes in prevalence and association with atopic dermatitis. Contact Dermatitis 2018;78(1):70–5.

64. Matthieu L, Dockx P. Discrepancy in patch test results with wool wax alcohols and Amerchol® L-101. Contact Dermatitis 1997;36(3):150–1.

65. Uter W, Schnuch A, Geier J. Contact sensitization to lanolin alcohols and Amerchol® L101 – analysis of IVDK data. Contact Dermatitis 2018;78(5):367–9.

66. Quenan S, Piletta P, Calza AM. Isothiazolinones: sensitizers not to miss in children. Pediatr Dermatol 2015;32(3):e86–8.

67. Castanedo-Tardana MP, Zug KA. Methylisothiazolinone. Dermatitis 2013; 24(1):2–6.

68. Yu SH, Sood A, Taylor JS. Patch testing for methylisothiazolinone and methylchloroisothiazolinone-methylisothiazolinone contact allergy. JAMA Dermatol 2016;152(1):67–72.

69. Schlichte MJ, Katta R. Methylisothiazolinone: an emergent allergen in common pediatric skin care products. Dermatol Res Pract 2014;2014:13256.

70. Goldenberg A, Lipp M, Jacob SE. Appropriate testing of isothiazolinones in children. Pediatr Dermatol 2017;34(2):138–43.

71. Christiansen MS, Agner T, Ebbehøj NE. Long-lasting allergic contact dermatitis caused by methylisothiazolinone in wall paint: a case report. Contact Dermatitis 2018;79(2):112–3.

72. Lundov MD, Kolarik B, Bossi R, et al. Emission of isothiazolinones from water-based paints. Environ Sci Technol 2014;48(12):6989–94.

73. Zhang AJ, Boyd AH, Asch S, et al. Allergic contact dermatitis to slime: the epidemic of isothiazolinone allergy encompasses school glue. Pediatr Dermatol 2019;36(1):e37–8.

74. Boyapati A, Tam M, Tate B, et al. Allergic contact dermatitis to methylisothiazolinone: exposure from baby wipes causing hand dermatitis. Australas J Dermatol 2013;54(4):264–7.

75. Kazandjieva J, Gergovska M, Darlenski R. Contact dermatitis in a child from methylchloroisothiazolinone and methylisothiazolinone in moist wipes. Pediatr Dermatol 2014;31(2):225–7.

76. Aerts O, Cattaert N, Lambert J, et al. Airborne and systemic dermatitis, mimicking atopic dermatitis, caused by methylisothiazolinone in a young child. Contact Dermatitis 2013;68(4):250–1.

77. Pessotti NS, Hafner M, Possa MS, et al. Allergic contact dermatitis to slime. An Bras Dermatol 2020;95(2):265–6.

78. Mainwaring W, Zhao J, Hunt R. Allergic contact dermatitis related to homemade slime: a case and review of the literature. Dermatol Online J 2019;25(4). 13030/qt7n06w0hg.

79. Isaksson M, Ale I, Andersen KE, et al. Patch testing with formaldehyde 2.0% (0.60 mg/cm2) detects more contact allergy to formaldehyde than 1.0%. Dermatitis 2019;30(6):342–6.

80. Flyvholm MA, Hall BM, Agner T, et al. Threshold for occluded formaldehyde patch test in formaldehyde-sensitive patients. Relationship to repeated open application test with a product containing formaldehyde releaser. Contact Dermatitis 1997;36(1):26–33.

81. Gruvberger B, Bruze M, Tammela M. Preservatives in moisturizers on the Swedish market. Acta Derm Venereol 1998;78(1):52–6.

82. Pontén A, Bruze M. Formaldehyde. Contact Dermatitis 2015;26(1):3–6.

83. DeKoven JG, Warshaw EM, Belsito DV, et al. North American contact dermatitis group patch test results 2013-2014. Dermatitis 2017;28(1):33–46.

84. Kundak S. Patch test results of contact sensitization in children without atopic dermatitis: a single tertiary center experience. Dermatitis 2020;31(2):153–6.

85. Moustafa D, Yu J De. Contact allergy to hydroperoxides of limonene and linalool in a pediatric population. J Am Acad Dermatol 2020;83(3):946–7.

86. de Groot A. Limonene Hydroperoxides. Dermatitis 2019;30(6):331–5.

87. de Groot A. Linalool Hydroperoxides. Dermatitis 2019;30(4):243–6.

88. Herman A, Darrigade AS, de Montjoye L, et al. Contact dermatitis caused by glucose sensors in diabetic children. Contact Dermatitis 2020;82(2):105–11.

89. Englert K, Ruedy K, Coffey J, et al. Skin and adhesive issues with continuous glucose monitors: a sticky situation. J Diabetes Sci Technol 2014;8(4):745–51.

90. Heinemann L, Kamann S. Adhesives used for diabetes medical devices: a neglected risk with serious consequences? J Diabetes Sci Technol 2016;10(6):1211–5.

91. Herman A, de Montjoye L, Tromme I, et al. Allergic contact dermatitis caused by medical devices for diabetes patients: a review. Contact Dermatitis 2018;79(6):331–5.

92. Herman A, Aerts O, Baeck M, et al. Allergic contact dermatitis caused by isobornyl acrylate in Freestyle® Libre, a newly introduced glucose sensor. Contact Dermatitis 2017;77(6):367–73.

93. Kamann S, Aerts O, Heinemann L. Further evidence of severe allergic contact dermatitis from isobornyl acrylate while using a continuous glucose monitoring system. J Diabetes Sci Technol 2018;12(3):630–3.

94. Aerts O, Herman A, Mowitz M, et al. Isobornyl Acrylate. Dermatitis 2020;31(1):4–12.

95. Darrigade AS, Raison-Peyron N, Courouge-Dorcier D, et al. The chemical acetophenone azine: an important cause of shin and foot dermatitis in children. J Eur Acad Dermatol Venereol 2020;34(2):e61–2.

96. Raison-Peyron N, Bergendorff O, Bourrain JL, et al. Acetophenone azine: a new allergen responsible for severe contact dermatitis from shin pads. Contact Dermatitis 2016;75(2):106–10.
97. Koumaki D, Bergendorff O, Bruze M, et al. Allergic contact dermatitis to shin pads in a hockey player: acetophenone is an emerging allergen. Dermatitis 2019;30(2):162–3.
98. Raison-Peyron N, Sasseville D. Acetophenone Azine. Dermatitis 2021;32(1):5–9.
99. Jacob SE, Brankov N, Kerr A. Diagnosis and management of allergic contact dermatitis in children: common allergens that can be easily missed. Curr Opin Pediatr 2017;29(4):443–7.
100. ACDS CAMP | American Contact Dermatitis Society (ACDS). Available at: https://www.contactderm.org/resources/acds-camp. Accessed August 31, 2020.
101. Scheman A, Hylwa-Deufel S, Jacob SE, et al. Alternatives for allergens in the 2018 american contact dermatitis society core series: report by the American Contact Alternatives Group. Dermatitis 2019;30(2):87–105.
102. Hill H, Goldenberg A, Golkar L, et al. Pre-Emptive Avoidance Strategy (P.E.A.S.)-addressing allergic contact dermatitis in pediatric populations. Expert Rev Clin Immunol 2016;12(5):551–61.
103. Brankov N, Jacob SE. Pre-emptive avoidance strategy 2016: update on pediatric contact dermatitis allergens. Expert Rev Clin Immunol 2017;13(2):93–5.

# Epidemics of Dermatitis

Mohsen Baghchechi, BS[a], Alina Goldenberg, MD, MAS[b],
Sharon E. Jacob, MD[a,c],*

## KEYWORDS

- Contact dermatitis • Epidemics • Dillarstone effect • Allergens • Patch testing

## KEY POINTS

- Epidemics are a result of a sudden increase in cases of a disease state from baseline over a specified time period.
- The Dillarstone effect describes the potential for development of a contact dermatitis epidemic in the 2- to 3-year wake of mass introduction of an alternative preservative to market.
- Diagnostic patch testing provides insight to allergen prevalence rates and the potential opportunity to detect epidemics by applying prevalence data.

## BACKGROUND
### Defining an Epidemic

An epidemic describes a sudden increase in cases of a disease process across a geographic region.[1] Although a disease may be intrinsically in constant presence—endemic, an acute increase in cases warrants epidemiologic investigation. The origin of the term *epidemic* dates back to ancient Greece, with Hippocrates observing abrupt population disease processes.[2] Historically, infectious agents are considered as prime causes of epidemics; however, noninfectious diseases including diabetes mellitus type 2, obesity, opioid abuse, and even allergic contact dermatitis (ACD) have been shown to have increasing prevalence rates in epidemic proportions. Although shared geography plays a role in epidemics, common attributes among a population including occupation and environmental exposure are also markedly important.[3]

### Factors Influencing a Surge

A multitude of factors play an interconnected role in the development of an epidemic surge, such as an increased presence of a primary causative agent, whether microbiological or environmental (eg, nickel, chromium), and increased

[a] University of California, Riverside, School of Medicine, 92521 UCR Botanic Gardens Road, Riverside, CA 92507, USA; [b] Dermatologist Medical Group of North County, 11943 EL Camino Real #220, San Diego, CA 92130, USA; [c] Veterans Health Administration, Loma Linda, 11210 Benton Street, Loma Linda, CA 92354, USA
* Corresponding author.
*E-mail address:* sjacob@contactderm.net

Immunol Allergy Clin N Am 41 (2021) 409–421
https://doi.org/10.1016/j.iac.2021.04.005
0889-8561/21/© 2021 Elsevier Inc. All rights reserved.
immunology.theclinics.com

chance of exposure to a population.[1] The duration of exposure to the causative agent or infection, along with an increased dose-dependent contact, is important in influencing epidemic surges.[4] Furthermore, an increase in susceptibility of individuals in a population, whether through migration or genetic susceptibility, may be the catalyst for an epidemic.[5,6]

### Factors Influencing Containment

Prevention remains the mainstay in epidemic containment and control.[7] Understanding and identifying at-risk individuals, for example, through primary prevention in the form of vaccinations or avoidance of environmental exposure, may help to curb case transmission or induction in an affected population.[8,9] It is important to recognize the fundamental role public health initiatives can play in the containment of both communicable and noncommunicable epidemics.[8,10]

## THE EPIDEMIC OF CONTACT DERMATITIS

Contact dermatitis is a highly prevalent dermatologic condition with considerable morbidity, affecting approximately 15% to 20% of the general population, including more than 4.4 million children in the United States (US).[11,12] In 2013, it was estimated that contact dermatitis roughly costs the US more than $1.5 billion in medical expenditure.[13] As a significant burden of occupational disease, contact dermatitis extends into the workforce with substantial losses for both employers and employees.

ACD leads to palpable morbidity and distress in the individuals expressing the disease. It often presents with intractable and debilitating dermatitis, which in occupational ACD has the potential to be career ending. Those working in wet-work fields such as hair dressing, beauticians, food preparation services, and those exposed to industrial chemicals are at increased risk, due to high frequency exposure to sensitizing agents on a skin barrier damaged by wet work. Of importance, wet work serves as an example of how low-grade irritant exposures can manifest in physical dysfunction and increased allergy susceptibility, paralleling a genetic predisposition seen in those with atopic dermatitis.[14,15] Because of the continuous and chronic exposure to a multitude of allergens within a wet environment, these workers maintain a high risk of developing allergies to even low-potency chemicals, in parallel to how atopic children are intrinsically more susceptible to developing ACD due to genetically impaired skin barriers.[16]

Children and infants may be at a particular risk for "early" sensitization if they have concomitant barrier dysfunction from underlying atopy. An impaired and permeable skin barrier allows for enhanced skin irritability with deeper dermal penetration of allergens.[17] A caveat to this has been reported in the literature, where allergens that are initially exposed to mucosa generate tolerance, rather than allergy, such as with early introduction of peanuts to children's diets has led to a decrease in peanut allergy worldwide.[18] Also, Mortz and colleagues determined that within a large childhood cohort there was a reduction in nickel allergy prevalence among girls with pierced who that had dental braces placed before piercing, further suggesting protection from early oral nickel exposure.[19] Historically, it was thought that the child's naïve immune system reduced the risk of delayed hypersensitivity compared with adults who have increased lifetime risk due to sustained encounters to allergens. In the last 2 decades, however, multiple studies have found sensitization rates comparable to adults in asymptomatic children aged 1 to 5 years, ranging from 13% to 24%.[12,20,21] The impact of childhood sensitization, given the extended lifetime risk of disease expression, is profound.

## THE METALS ALLERGIC CONTACT DERMITITIS EPIDEMIC

Chromium has been found responsible for ACD in occupations that handle cement. It has been shown that construction workers exposed to hexavalent chromium-based cement had sensitizing rates greater than 10%, whereas the allergy rate for workers exposed to reduced chromium is approximately 1%. The nonreduced hexavalent chromium can be reduced with the introduction of iron sulfate to a trivalent form that is water-insoluble and therefore innocuous to the skin-less sensitizing and a lower risk of developing ACD.[22,23] Since the 1980s, Denmark and the European Union (EU) have systematically added ferrous sulfate to cement to decrease its allergenic potential leading to a one-third decrease in levels of chromium sensitization; however, no such intervention exists in the US.[24] One of the reasons for resistance to this implementation among US manufacturers is that it is estimated that it would increase cement production costs by 1% to 1.5%, on top of the current projected $264 million cost per year in materials (Rycroft and colleagues, 2001).[25]

Over a century passed between the discovery of nickel in 1751 and the recognition of the first nickel-induced ACD case, published in Germany.[5,26] Thereafter, multiple outbreaks of contact dermatitis within the US have appeared in the literature, such as the electroplating industrial workers in the 1920s and an aggregation of cases in the 1930s relating to nickel in wearable items, such as sock suspenders.[5] The most sustained source of primary sensitization for the nickel epidemic over the last 3 decades has been body piercing and adornment. Schuttelaar and colleagues determined that within a European population those individuals with multiple piercings had increased prevalence of nickel sensitization.[27] Nickel-induced ACD secondary to piercings may be misdiagnosed as infections such as cellulitis and perichondritis, resulting in failure to address the underlying cause.[28] Over time, regulatory bodies in Europe moved to limit exposure of nickel within body piercings, starting with limiting nickel to less than 0.05% during the epithelialization in 1994. Within the US, avoidance strategies and replacing piercing jewelry with surgical steel or titanium are beneficial.[28]

Of note, reports of Ni-ACD to electronics (eg, watches, mobile phones, and tablets) started to emerge in the late 90s and have now been a significant source for well over a decade.[29] Of importance, several occupational sources to high-release nickel, such as scissors, keys, metallic tools, chairs, and coins, are also well-established sources in schools that could potentially sensitize children.[30] With early sensitization in childhood, there remains a looming risk of future occupational ACD during adulthood and even increased risk to medically necessary nickel containing devices (eg, orthopedic hardware, implantable cardiac devices, and dental alloys) in the future.[31]

The EU took meaningful steps to thwart this epidemic in the mid 1990s by introducing legislation to limit exposure to high-nickel release items that contacted skin, as approximately 15% to 30% of the population was found to be nickel sensitized. This legislation led to significant reductions in sensitizations in Europe, with 10% to 15% decrease seen since implementation.[32–34] It is important to note that even with the significant reduction in sensitization, nickel allergy remains prevalent. Schnuch and colleagues reported that among young German women, sensitization rates have stabilized at around 10% to 20% since the introduction of legislation in 1994.[35]

This has led epidemiologists to examine the factors contributing to the epidemic. For one, increased vigilance for additional exposure sources became paramount. Fenner and colleagues completed a systematic review of the literature and found multiple toys including putty, slime, bicycles, and electronics as a source of nickel-induced ACD in children.[36] Both an iPad (Apple Inc, Cupertino, CA, USA) and Xbox controller (Microsoft Corp, Redmond, WA, USA) were reported to cause nickel sensitization.[37,38]

The inexpensive dimethylglyoxime (DMG) test has long been used to quantify nickel release. The test takes advantage of the chelating reaction between nickel and DMG, allowing providers to simply deliver several drops of 1% DMG to a cotton tip applicator followed by rubbing the item in question. If the applicator turns pink, the test is considered positive. Thyssen and colleagues reports that the DMG test has a sensitivity and specificity of 59.3% and 97.5%, respectively, meaning the true prevalence may be underestimated.[39] In 1998, the European Committee for Standardization (ECS) developed the EN1811 directive as a nickel reference test to estimate nickel release designed to identify and label items that exceed 0.5um/cm$^2$ per week. This standardized synthetic sweat study is completed following immersion of the suspected item within artificial sweat (deionized water, sodium chloride 0.5%, lactic acid 0.1%, urea 0.1%, pH 6.5) and allowed to soak for 168 hours. Finally, analysis of nickel from the synthetic sweat was performed using plasma optical emission spectroscopy. The EN1811 assessment has a greater accuracy in detecting nickel release compared with DMG. With that said, the delay in test results, risk of damage to the item in question, and expense are all potential downsides to consider. In 2002, the ECS developed the EN12421 assessment that uses DMG for a quick and accurate screening tool that has the added benefit of prolonged exposure results.[39] It is of importance to define prolonged nickel exposure, as longer exposure times significantly increase risk of sensitization. In 2014, the European Chemical Agency defined prolonged nickel exposure as 10 minutes on 3 or more occasions within 2 weeks or 30 minutes on one or more instances in a 2-week period of time.[40]

The US has yet to implement similar regulations, leading to a continued epidemic of nickel-induced contact dermatitis, as nickel sensitization prevalence continues to increase in North America, as they did in Europe over 2 decades ago.[8,41] The American Academy of Pediatrics (AAP) recently issued a health policy and advisory position statement aiming to identify nickel contact sources and treat and avoid exposures while advocating for legislative changes in advancing manufacturing safety standards as have been implemented in the EU.[42] Considering the ubiquitous nature of nickel among commonly encountered materials, and the risk of profound ACD following sensitization, advocacy for sensitization prevention remains key. Specific recommendations by the AAP include advocating for a restriction of weekly release of nickel to 0.5ug/cm$^2$. Providers are also encouraged to counsel youths with high risk of allergy to avoid body piercings altogether or switch to surgical steel– or titanium-based products.

## THE INCREASE AND DECREASE OF PRESERVATIVES

Two preservative chemicals—methylchloroisothiazolinone (MCI) and methylisothiazolinone (MI)—have both been shown to have caused global contact dermatitis epidemics.[43] MCI was added to the market as a preservative in cosmetic products in the 1970s. Alternatively, it was also used in disinfectants, paints, detergent shampoos, and air conditioning systems. The popularity of the preservative stemmed from its dual bactericidal and fungicidal properties, which allowed for replacing of the harmful parabens and formaldehyde compounds. It was thought that the chlorinated group of MCI contained the highly allergenic component by forming a reactive intermediate.[44] To retain the antimicrobial effect and reduce the risk of sensitization to MCI, a formulation of a 3:1 MCI/MI mixture was introduced to market in 1977 under the trademark Kathon CG (Dow Chemical, Midland, MI, USA). By the mid-1980s the first ACD outbreak linked to MCI/MI was noted by the public health authorities. Quickly, this developed into an MCI/MI epidemic, reaching sensitization rates up to 5% of the population.[45]

Because the MCI/MI formulation remained a significant sensitizer in both pediatric and adult populations, MCI was limited in 2000 and led to the development of standalone MI preservative being approved in both industrial and cosmetic use by 2000 and 2005, respectively (**Table 1**).[46] To assure biocidal efficacy, MI concentrations were increased to match that of the MCI/MI preservative.[47]

The subsequent increase in permitted MI concentrations led to the beginnings of an epidemic identified in 2004.[48] The American Contact Dermatitis Society (ACDS) went on to name MI the 2013 contact allergen of the year.[49] Several largescale European studies note the MI sensitization rate at approximately 0.5% to 6% among the general population.[50] Interestingly, studies originating from Southern Europe showed significantly greater sensitization rates ranging from 7.2% to 19.6%.[51] A study by Dusefante and colleagues followed an Italian population over 20 years and reported a prevalence of MI sensitization at 5.47% among those younger than 25 years.[52] Another study by the North American Contact Dermatitis Group (NACDG) reported the prevalence of sensitivity to either MCI/MI or standalone MI at a staggering rate of 11.9% across North America.[53] One study investigated the discovery of MCI-/MI-induced ACD among water bottle plant workers, illustrating the implications this allergen has within the workforce.[54] Patch test standard substrates have been evidence tested and developed to detect MI/MCI at concentrations of 200 ppm, to avoid false-negative reactions in sensitized individuals.[55] A study by Engfeldt and colleagues reported a significant increase in the allergy detection rate from 3.7% to 5.6% for MCI/MI when testing with the 200 ppm standard substrate, rather than at 100 ppm.[56] Furthermore, it has been determined that detection of MI alone is greatly improved when testing is done at 2000 ppm.[57]

Of special note, the pediatric population remains highly vulnerable to sensitization by MI considering the inclusion of MI in a high number of products intended for pediatric use, cleansing wipes, sunscreens, shampoos, moisturizers, and bubble

**Table 1**
**Utilization of the preservative methylisothiazolinone**

| Exposure Source | Cosmetics | Household | Occupation/ Industry |
|---|---|---|---|
| Examples | Shampoo (53%) | Dishwashing soap (64%) | Paints |
| | Conditioner (45%) | Household cleaner (47%) | Glues |
| | Facewash | Laundry additives/ | Eyeglass frames |
| | Mouthwash | softener (30%) | Wound vacuum |
| | Handwash | Surface disinfectants (27%) | pump |
| | Deodorant | Laundry detergent (13%) | Roofing material |
| | Wet wipes | Glass cleaner | Printer ink |
| | Hair dyes (43%) | | Ultrasound gel |
| | Moisturizer (82%) | | Cutting fluid |
| | Shaving products (78%) | | Coolants |
| | Sunscreen (71%) | | |
| | Sodium hyaluronate | | |
| | Makeup remover | | |
| | Bubble baths | | |
| References | | | |

Exposure sources with a corresponding percentage indicate the percentage of products that contained MI based on a 2013 analysis of products from the CAMP database by the American Contact Dermatitis Society (Scheman and Severson, 2016).
Utilization of the preservative methylisothiazolinone (MI) among industrial, household, and cosmetic products.

baths.[58,59] A case report by Chang and colleagues describes ACD in the diaper region of infants following use of MI cleansing wipes, with complete resolution following discontinuation of the product.[60] Another study described a case of hand dermatitis in a parent using wet wipes containing MI.[61]

The ACD epidemics to preservatives are the result of a recognizable sequence, starting with introduction of potential allergens into manufactured products, followed by increased utilization of these products by the populous, leading to increased sensitization rates and the development of exponentially elevated cases of ACD, followed by public outcry resulting in removal of the allergen and replacement with an alternative, and then increased incidence of ACD to the alternative—all summarized by the phenomenon titled *The Dillarstone effect*.[62]

## THE DILLARSTONE EFFECT

Warnings of the potential harm caused by compounds from the isothiazolinone family are found in the literature dating back to the early 1990s.[63] In 1997, Alan Dillarstone described a phenomenon in which newly introduced preservatives, marketed as alternatives to identified allergenic preservatives, would enter the market seemingly absolvent of initial negative allergic effect, only to surface after a latent period of 2 to 3 years, and later be followed by the development of a new contact dermatitis epidemic.[62]

A 24-year retrospective preservative allergy study in Denmark set out to challenge the Dillarstone effect.[39] The study confirmed that positive patch test prevalence to preservatives decreased for agents that had been banned and removed from the market, whereas others still being used continued to have prevalent sensitizations.[39] Furthermore, agents for which there was increased use and application were shown to be associated with increasing prevalence rates, confirming the Dillarstone effect.

Sunscreen is another globally used product and example illustrating the Dillarstone effect over the past century. Because the first ultraviolet (UV) filter was patented in 1928 in the US, organic UV filters have been responsible for multiple reports of ACD, as well as a subtype known as photoallergic ACD.[64] These organic UV filters effectively absorb UV wavelengths through their aromatic structure that aids in electron resonance stability.[64] However, marketed UV filters are only able to absorb specific wavelengths of light, and thus topical sunscreens require multiple filters to cover a broader spectrum. Para-aminobenzoic acid (PABA) derivatives and cinnamates were some of the earliest filters created to prevent UV-B light absorption. As more reports of ACD secondary to PABA and cinnamate derivatives emerged, coupled with research suggesting UV-A radiation is indeed harmful, manufacturers responded by reducing the use of PABA and developing and introducing a new family of organic filters known as the benzophenones. Soon thereafter, concern was raised that benzophenone-3, oxybenzone, and benzophenone-4 reportedly caused marked rates of ACD in users.[65] Multiple epidemiologic reports were published describing high rates of positive patch testing to the benzophenone filters were associated with sunscreens and various other products including printer ink, toiletries, and most recently industrial work.[65–68] Following a 10-year retrospective analysis, Warshaw and colleagues notes that greater than 70% of patients with a reported allergy to sunscreen had a benzophenone-3 positive patch test.[69] In response to the continued ACD prevalence, the Food and Drug Administration set measures to limit benzophenone-3 and 4 to maximum concentrations of 6% and 10%, respectively.[65]

Thus, Dillarstone's observation underscores the importance of surveillance as an integral tool to identify an ACD epidemic and suggests that banning allergenic substances is often unwarranted, as it results in a new epidemic to the substituted chemical. Acknowledging the allergenic potential of various substances allows for epidemic studies to identify and track potential allergens that should be removed from the market to reduce sensitization rates. Vigilant surveillance paired with confirmatory diagnostic patch testing remains the most effective mechanism to contain in the ACD epidemic.

## THE ROLE OF SURVEILLANCE

It is often difficult for a patient to isolate the exact causative agent, given that the average person comes into contact with a myriad of chemicals daily and that the pathophysiological mechanism of the disease inherently has a delayed presentation from the time of exposure. For this reason, epicutaneous patch testing is the gold standard in identifying potential allergen sensitizations in individuals who suffer from ACD.[70,71] With more than 4000 chemicals in use today and an ever-increasing number of novel chemicals introduced into manufactured products, the risk of continued contact dermatitis epidemics increases.[72]

Patch testing is the primary method of collecting epidemiologic prevalence of contact dermatitis. An international collaboration by the International Contact Dermatitis Research Group (ICDRG), formed in 1966, developed a standard 20 panel patch test of common worldwide allergens in 1997, followed by an additional 12 panel expansion in 2011.[73–75] The ICDRG considers recommending a hapten for inclusion in patch testing if there is a 0.5% to 1% rate of allergy in tested individuals.

The NACDG developed a 65-allergen panel to survey patients referred for patch testing.[76] The results from the most recently published study period 2015 to 2017 demonstrated that greater than 50% of the referred patients met the criteria for the diagnosis of ACD using an updated 70-allergen panel.[77] Similarly, the American Contact Dermatitis Society (ACDS) proposed an 80-core allergen series in 2009.[78] The increased panel size allows for greater breadth in detection and may be fine-tuned depending on the provider's preferences.[79] The ACDS went on to develop the Contact Allergen Management Program (CAMP), which is designed to help patients avoid known allergens and seek alternatives through a comprehensive and evolving database.[80] Another key element of CAMP is the ability to use the allergen database to modify and adapt the ACDS core panel in the years to come.

Before 2008, there were no large multicenter retrospective patch test studies nor pediatric research collaboratives. In 2014, the Pediatric Contact Dermatitis Registry was introduced, and within the first year over 250 providers across the US reported performing patch testing on children.[81] The group noted an alarming finding that US children were confirmed to have equivalent sensitization rates to US adults on a large scale.[82] The data also revealed important trends in patch testing practices and access and highlighted the considerable need for continued surveillance through appropriate use of patch testing and data sharing.[83] When epidemics to allergens are identified, exposures should be modified and changed promptly.

## PREEMPTIVE AVOIDANCE STRATEGIES

Avoidance of allergens remains the primary treatment and preventative measure against a contact dermatitis epidemic. The utilization of a preemptive avoidance strategies (P.E.A.S.) has been shown to be effective in cases "too rashy to patch test," for those with limited access to evaluative patch testing and for those with history of atopy.[84] At-risk groups with decreased access to testing, such as children with concomitant eczema, may be of particular benefit from P.E.A.S.[85] There are thousands of potential chemical sensitizers that individuals come into contact with each day. That said, there is a core group of allergens to which the public has been consistently exposed to for decades, making these the more likely sources of hypersensitivity among the general population.[86] By preferentially preemptively avoiding these high yield allergens, the individuals sensitized to them demonstrate improvement of their dermatitis will improve.[82] Readily available listings of potential sources of allergens with corresponding prevalence from recent epidemiologic studies are the basis behind the P.E.A.S. strategy for safer alternatives and may be found on the Dermatitis Academy (DA) Web site. The DA is a free online resource that encompasses education, outreach, and support for patients and providers. The Web site offers access to many user-friendly educational pamphlets and videos on allergens, recommendations on avoidance measures, and a centralized source of top-rated mobile apps to help families living with ACD.

## THE ROLE OF ACCESS TO ALTERNATIVES

Online databases exist for providers seeking alternative products that do not contain ingredients to which their patients have demonstrated clinically relevant positive patch test reactions. For example, CAMP replaced the Contact Allergen Replacement Database as the database of allergenic products for the ACDS.[71,87] This online platform allows the provider to input particular patient-specific allergens, check for cross-reactors, and provide a list of skincare products devoid of the patient's known allergens.[88] Members of the ACDS are able to provide individual patients a unique identifier with their CAMP alternative products list following patch testing. Patients can then use the CAMP mobile app feature to access information on the go and even digitally scan products for instant feedback. Thus, consistent avoidance of allergens with the assistance of the aforementioned resources can assist in keeping contact dermatitis from flaring.

## SUMMARY

Contact dermatitis remains a globally prevalent disease that will continue to expand as long as current allergens continue to be used and new allergens are introduced into the market. A literature search over the past 70 years has highlighted multiple contact dermatitis epidemics from heavy metals to preservative ingredients found in everyday products. A closer look at epidemics in 1997 led to the development of the "Dillarstone effect," describing the phenomenon where new epidemics are primed to increase approximately 3 years following mass introduction of alternative preservative agents. Vigilant surveillance through diagnostic patch remains key in containing the ACD epidemic. Because contact dermatitis continues to cause marked morbidity for many individuals, additional research and involvement of manufacturing and legislative changes, along with public health initiates, are needed to curb this epidemic.

## CLINICS CARE POINTS

- If novel allergens are identified, consider reporting for epidemiologic tracing, rather than proposing an allergen ban, as to avoid perpetuating the Dillarstone effect.
- If ACD is suspected, immediately discontinue aggravating product and refer patient to use preemptive strategies and enroll in online mobile contact allergen programs designed to reduce allergen exposure (eg, CAMP).
- In children with underlying atopy, have a high index of suspicion for ACD and implement preventative strategies early.

- If the underlying allergen resulting in ACD remains elusive, perform epicutaneous patch testing, which remains the gold standard in identifying potential allergen sensitization.

## DISCLOSURE

The authors have nothing to disclose. S.E. Jacob owns Dermatitis Academy.

## REFERENCES

1. Center for Disease Control and Prevention. Principles of Epidemiology in Public Health Practice, Third Edition An Introduction to Applied Epidemiology and Biostatistics: Level of Disease. 2012. Available at: https://www.cdc.gov/csels/dsepd/ss1978/lesson1/section11.html. [Accessed 20 June 2020].
2. Martin PM, Martin-Granel E. 2,500-year evolution of the term epidemic. Emerg Infect Dis 2006;12(6):976–80.
3. Orbann C, Sattenspiel L, Miller E, et al. Defining epidemics in computer simulation models: How do definitions influence conclusions? Epidemics 2017;19:24–32.
4. Thyssen JP, Johansen JD, Menné T. Contact allergy epidemics and their controls. Contact Dermatitis 2007;56(4):185–95.
5. Mackintosh DR, Stewart GT. A mathematical model of a heroin epidemic: implications for control policies. J Epidemiol Community Health 1979;33(4):299–304.
6. Friedmann PS, Sanchez-Elsner T, Schnuch A. Genetic factors in susceptibility to contact sensitivity. Contact Dermatitis 2015;72(5):263–74.
7. Peng XL, Xu XJ, Small M, et al. Prevention of infectious diseases by public vaccination and individual protection. J Math Biol 2016;73(6–7):1561–94.
8. Silverberg NB, Pelletier JL, Jacob SE, et al, Section on Dermatology, Section on Allergy And Immunology. Nickel Allergic Contact Dermatitis: Identification, Treatment, and Prevention. Pediatrics 2020;145(5):e20200628.
9. Andersen KE. Occupational issues of allergic contact dermatitis. Int Arch Occup Environ Health 2003;76(5):347–50.
10. Saklayen MG. The global epidemic of the metabolic syndrome. Curr Hypertens Rep 2018;20(2):12.
11. Peiser M, Tralau T, Heidler J, et al. Allergic contact dermatitis: epidemiology, molecular mechanisms, in vitro methods and regulatory aspects. Current knowledge assembled at an international workshop at BfR, Germany. Cell Mol Life Sci 2012;69(5):763–81.
12. Borok J, Matiz C, Goldenberg A, et al. Contact Dermatitis in Atopic Dermatitis Children-Past, Present, and Future. Clin Rev Allergy Immunol 2019;56(1):86–98.
13. Lim HW, Collins SAB, Resneck JS Jr, et al. The burden of skin disease in the United States. J Am Acad Dermatol 2017;76(5):958–72.e2.
14. Nedorost ST. Allergic contact sensitization in healthy skin differs from sensitization in chronic dermatitis: atopic, occupational wet work, and stasis dermatitis. Dermatol Clin 2020;38(3):301–8.
15. Visser MJ, Landeck L, Campbell LE, et al. Impact of atopic dermatitis and loss-of-function mutations in the filaggrin gene on the development of occupational irritant contact dermatitis. Br J Dermatol 2013;168(2):326–32.
16. Kohli N, Nedorost S. Inflamed skin predisposes to sensitization to less potent allergens. J Am Acad Dermatol 2016;75(2):312–7.e1.
17. Proksch E, Brasch J. Abnormal epidermal barrier in the pathogenesis of contact dermatitis. Clin Dermatol 2012;30(3):335–44.

18. White JM, Goon AT, Jowsey IR, et al. Oral tolerance to contact allergens: a common occurrence? A review. Contact Dermatitis 2007;56(5):247–54.
19. Mortz CG, Lauritsen JM, Bindslev-Jensen C, et al. Nickel sensitization in adolescents and association with ear piercing, use of dental braces and hand eczema. The Odense Adolescence Cohort Study on Atopic Diseases and Dermatitis (TOACS). Acta Derm Venereol 2002;82(5):359–64.
20. Bruckner AL, Weston WL, Morelli JG. Does sensitization to contact allergens begin in infancy? Pediatrics 2000;105(1):e3.
21. Barros MA, Baptista A, Correia TM, et al. Patch testing in children: a study of 562 schoolchildren. Contact Dermatitis 1991;25(3):156–9.
22. Fregert S, Gruvberger B, Sandahl E. Reduction of chromate in cement by iron sulfate. Contact Dermatitis 1979;5(1):39–42.
23. Valverde JL, Lobato J, Fernandez I, et al. Ferrous sulphate mono and heptahydrate reduction of hexavalent chromium in cement: effectiveness and storability. Mater Construcc 2005;55(279):39–52.
24. Roto P, Sainio H, Reunala T, et al. Addition of ferrous sulfate to cement and risk of chromium dermatitis among construction workers. Contact Dermatitis 1996;34(1): 43–50.
25. Rycroft RJG, Menne T, Frosch PJ, et al. Textbook of contact dermatitis. third edition. Berlin, Heidelberg: Springer-Verlag; 2001. p. 442.
26. Menne T, Maibach HI. Nickel allergic contact dermatitis: a review. J Am Coll Toxicol 1989;8(7):1271–3.
27. Schuttelaar MLA, Ofenloch RF, Bruze M, et al. Prevalence of contact allergy to metals in the European general population with a focus on nickel and piercings: The EDEN Fragrance Study. Contact Dermatitis 2018;79(1):1–9.
28. Ivey LA, Limone BA, Jacob SE. Approach to the jewelry aficionado. Pediatr Dermatol 2018;35(2):274–5.
29. Roberts H, Tate B. Nickel allergy presenting as mobile phone contact dermatitis. Australas J Dermatol 2010;51(1):23–5.
30. Tuchman M, Silverberg JI, Jacob SE, et al. Nickel contact dermatitis in children. Clin Dermatol 2015;33(3):320–6.
31. Kettelarij JA, Lidén C, Axén E, et al. Cobalt, nickel and chromium release from dental tools and alloys. Contact Dermatitis 2014;70(1):3–10.
32. Garg S, Thyssen JP, Uter W, et al. Nickel allergy following European Union regulation in Denmark, Germany, Italy and the U.K. Br J Dermatol 2013;169(4):854–8.
33. Thyssen JP, Engkilde K, Lundov MD, et al. Temporal trends of preservative allergy in Denmark (1985-2008). Contact Dermatitis 2010;62(2):102–8.
34. Johansen Jd, Menné T, Christophersen J, et al. Changes in the pattern of sensitization to common contact allergens in denmark between 1985-86 and 1997-98, with a special view to the effect of preventive strategies. Br J Dermatol 2000; 142(3):490–5.
35. Schnuch A, Wolter J, Geier J, et al. Nickel allergy is still frequent in young German females - probably because of insufficient protection from nickel-releasing objects. Contact Dermatitis 2011;64(3):142–50.
36. Fenner J, Hadi A, Yeh L, et al. Hidden risks in toys: a systematic review of pediatric toy contact dermatitis. Contact Dermatitis 2020;82(5):265–71.
37. Jacob SE, Admani S. iPad–increasing nickel exposure in children. Pediatrics 2014;134(2):e580–2.
38. Jacob SE. Xbox–a source of nickel exposure in children. Pediatr Dermatol 2014; 31(1):115–6.

39. Thyssen JP, Uter W, McFadden J, et al. The EU Nickel Directive revisited–future steps towards better protection against nickel allergy. Contact Dermatitis 2011; 64(3):121–5.
40. Nixon RL, Higgins CL, Maor D, et al. Does clinical testing support the current guidance definition of prolonged contact for nickel allergy? Contact Dermatitis 2018;79(6):356–64.
41. Rietschel RL, Fowler JF, Warshaw EM, et al. Detection of nickel sensitivity has increased in North American patch-test patients. Dermatitis 2008;19(1):16–9.
42. Pelletier J, Jacob SE, Silverberg NB. Policy helps identify, treat, prevent nickel allergy contact dermatitis. AAP News and Journals. 2020. Available at: https://pediatrics.aappublications.org/content/early/2020/04/23/peds.2020-0628. Accessed September 12, 2020.
43. Lundov MD, Thyssen JP, Zachariae C, et al. Prevalence and cause of methylisothiazolinone contact allergy. Contact Dermatitis 2010;63(3):164–7.
44. Alexander BR. An assessment of the comparative sensitization potential of some common isothiazolinones. Contact Dermatitis 2002;46(4):191–6.
45. Wilkinson JD, Shaw S, Andersen KE, et al. Monitoring levels of preservative sensitivity in Europe. A 10-year overview (1991-2000). Contact Dermatitis 2002;46(4): 207–10.
46. Yim E, Baquerizo Nole KL, Tosti A. Contact dermatitis caused by preservatives. Dermatitis 2014;25:215–31.
47. Geier J, Lessmann H, Schnuch A, et al. Recent increase in allergic reactions to methylchloroisothiazolinone/methylisothiazolinone: is methylisothiazolinone the culprit? Contact Dermatitis 2012;67(6):334–41.
48. García-Gavín J, Vansina S, Kerre S, et al. Methylisothiazolinone, an emerging allergen in cosmetics? Contact Dermatitis 2010;63(2):96–101.
49. Yu SH, Sood A, Taylor JS. Patch testing for methylisothiazolinone and methylchloroisothiazolinone-methylisothiazolinone contact allergy. JAMA Dermatol 2016;152(1):67–72.
50. Puangpet P, Chawarung A, McFadden JP. Methylchloroisothiazolinone/Methylisothiazolinone and methylisothiazolinone allergy. Dermatitis 2015;26(2):99–102.
51. Herman A, Aerts O, de Montjoye L, et al. Isothiazolinone derivatives and allergic contact dermatitis: a review and update. J Eur Acad Dermatol Venereol 2019; 33(2):267–76.
52. Dusefante A, Mauro M, Belloni Fortina A, et al. Contact allergy to methylchloroisothiazolinone/methylisothiazolinone in north-eastern Italy: a temporal trend from 1996 to 2016. J Eur Acad Dermatol Venereol 2019;33(5):912–7.
53. Zirwas MJ, Hamann D, Warshaw EM, et al. Epidemic of isothiazolinone allergy in North America: prevalence data from the North American contact dermatitis group, 2013-2014. Dermatitis 2017;28(3):204–9.
54. Hollins LC, Hallock K, Disse M, et al. Occupationally induced allergic contact dermatitis to methylchloroisothiazolinone/methylisothiazolinone among water bottle plant workers. Dermatitis 2020;31(4):265–7.
55. Leiva-Salinas M, Frances L, Marin-Cabanas I, et al. Methylchloroisothiazolinone/ methylisothiazolinone and methylisothiazolinone allergies can be detected by 200 ppm of methylchloroisothiazolinone/methylisothiazolinone patch test concentration. Dermatitis 2014;25(3):130–4.
56. Engfeldt M, Ale I, Andersen KE, et al. Multicenter patch testing with methylchloroisothizoline/methylisothiazolinone in 100 and 200 ppm within the international contact dermatitis research group. Dermatitis 2017;28(3):215–8.

57. Wilford JE, de Gannes GC. Methylisothiazolinone contact allergy prevalence in Western Canada: increased detection with 2000 ppm patch test allergen. J Cutan Med Surg 2017;21(3):207–10.
58. Goldenberg A, Lipp M, Jacob SE. Appropriate testing of isothiazolinones in children. Pediatr Dermatol 2017;34(2):138–43.
59. Quenan S, Piletta P, Calza AM. Isothiazolinones: sensitizers not to miss in children. Pediatr Dermatol 2015;32(3):e86–8.
60. Chang MW, Nakrani R. Six children with allergic contact dermatitis to methylisothiazolinone in wet wipes (baby wipes). Pediatrics 2014;133(2):e434–8.
61. Boyapati A, Tam M, Tate B, et al. Allergic contact dermatitis to methylisothiazolinone: exposure from baby wipes causing hand dermatitis. Australas J Dermatol 2013;54(4):264–7.
62. Dillarstone A. Cosmetic preservatives. Letter to the Editor. Contact Dermatitis 1997;37:190.
63. Dillarstone A. 1,2-benzisothiazolin-3-one. Contact Dermatitis 1993;28(1):53.
64. Bens G. Sunscreens. Adv Exp Med Biol 2014;810:429–63.
65. Heurung AR, Raju SI, Warshaw EM. Benzophenones [published correction appears in Dermatitis. 2014 Mar-Apr;25(2):92-5]. Dermatitis 2014;25(1):3–10.
66. Caruana DM, McPherson T, Cooper S. Allergic contact dermatitis caused by benzophenone-4 in a printer. Contact Dermatitis 2011;64:183–4.
67. Fisher AA. Sunscreen dermatitis: part III—the benzophenones. Cutis 1992;50: 331–2.
68. Scheman A, Jacob S, Katta R, et al. Part 4 of a 4-part series miscellaneous products: trends and alternatives in deodorants, antiperspirants, sunblocks, shaving products, powders, and wipes: data from the American Contact Alternatives Group. J Clin Aesthet Dermatol 2011;4(10):36–9.
69. Warshaw EM, Wang MZ, Maibach HI, et al. Patch test reactions associated with sunscreen products and the importance of testing to an expanded series: retrospective analysis of North American Contact Dermatitis Group data, 2001 to 2010. Dermatitis 2013;24:176–82.
70. Mowad CM, Anderson B, Scheinman P, et al. Allergic contact dermatitis: Patient diagnosis and evaluation. J Am Acad Dermatol 2016;74(6):1029–40.
71. Nassau S, Fonacier L. Allergic contact dermatitis. Med Clin North Am 2020; 104(1):61–76.
72. Mowad CM. Contact dermatitis: practice gaps and challenges. Dermatol Clin 2016;34(3):263–7.
73. Alikhan A, Cheng LS, Ale I, et al. Revised minimal baseline series of the International Contact Dermatitis Research Group: evidence-based approach. Dermatitis 2011;22(2):121–2.
74. Calnan CD, Fregert S, Magnusson B. The international contact dermatitis research group. Cutis 1976;18(5):708–10.
75. Isaksson M, Ale I, Andersen KE, et al. Revised baseline series of the international contact dermatitis [corrected] research group [published online ahead of print, 2020 Jan 3] [published correction appears in Dermatitis. 2020 Mar/Apr;31(2):166]. Dermatitis 2020;31(1):e5–7.
76. Cohen DE, Rao S, Brancaccio RR. Use of the North American Contact Dermatitis Group Standard 65-allergen series alone in the evaluation of allergic contact dermatitis: a series of 794 patients. Dermatitis 2008;19(3):137–41.
77. DeKoven JG, Warshaw EM, Zug KA, et al. North American Contact Dermatitis Group Patch Test Results: 2015-2016. Dermatitis 2018;29(6):297–309.

78. Lee J, Warshaw E, Zirwas MJ. Allergens in the American Contact Dermatitis Society Core Series. Clin Dermatol 2011;29(3):266–72.
79. Schalock PC, Dunnick CA, Nedorost S, et al. American Contact Dermatitis Society Core Allergen Series: 2017 Update. Dermatitis 2017;28(2):141–3.
80. Scheman A, Patel KR, Roszko K, et al. Relative prevalence of contact allergens in North America in 2018. Dermatitis 2020;31(2):112–21.
81. Jacob SE, McGowan M, Silverberg NB, et al. Pediatric contact dermatitis registry data on contact allergy in children with atopic dermatitis. JAMA Dermatol 2017; 153(8):765–70.
82. Goldenberg A, Mousdicas N, Silverberg N, et al. Pediatric contact dermatitis registry inaugural case data. Dermatitis 2016;27(5):293–302.
83. Jacob SE, Lipp MB, Suh E, et al. Practice patterns of dermatologists in the pediatric contact dermatitis registry. Pediatr Dermatol 2017;34(4):408–12.
84. Hill H, Goldenberg A, Golkar L, et al. Pre-Emptive Avoidance Strategy (P.E.A.S.) - addressing allergic contact dermatitis in pediatric populations. Expert Rev Clin Immunol 2016;12(5):551–61.
85. Brankov N, Jacob SE. Pre-emptive avoidance strategy 2016: update on pediatric contact dermatitis allergens. Expert Rev Clin Immunol 2017;13(2):93–5.
86. Militello G, Jacob SE, Crawford GH. Allergic contact dermatitis in children. Curr Opin Pediatr 2006;18(4):385–90.
87. Scheman A, Severson D. American contact dermatitis society contact allergy management program: an epidemiologic tool to determine relative prevalence of contact allergens. Dermatitis 2016;27(1):9–10.
88. Caperton C, Jacob SE. Improving post-patch-test education with the contact allergen replacement database. Dermatitis 2007;18(2):101–2.

# Laboratory Techniques for Identifying Causes of Allergic Dermatitis

Itai Chipinda, PhD[a], Stacey E. Anderson, PhD[b],*,
Paul D. Siegel, PhD[b]

## KEYWORDS

• Allergic contact dermatitis • Hazard identification • Patch test • Chemical analysis

## KEY POINTS

- Validated rapid and sensitive laboratory-based analyses are available to screen chemicals for sensitization potential.
- Laboratory-based chemical analyses can be used to confirm the presence of a patient's putative etiologic allergic contact dermatitis agent, identify unknown allergens, evaluate patch test quality, and test the quality of commercial chemical spot tests.
- Chemical analyses can be complex, time consuming, and costly, which may prohibit its use for routine patient care.

## HAZARD IDENTIFICATION
### Animal-Based Tests

Because of the environmental, occupational, and clinical significance of chemical sensitizers that induce allergic contact dermatitis (ACD), the use of rapid and sensitive methods for hazard identification is necessary. A human-based assay known as the human repeat insult patch test (HRIPT) has been used to confirm skin allergy; however, because of ethical concerns and alternate methods, the use of this assay has been eliminated in many countries.[1] Two guinea pig-based assays, the guinea pig maximization test (GPMT) and the Buehler assay, have been used to predict chemical sensitizers. These assays are recommended for use by the Organization for Economic Cooperation and Development (OECD) as test guideline (TG) 406.[2] The GPMT uses intradermal administration of a test chemical combined with or without Freund complete adjuvant followed by topical administration of the test chemical. Two weeks after topical dosing, the animals are challenged by patch test of the flank and the allergic reaction, on the skin is assessed to measure sensitization potential.[3] The Buehler

[a] Global Product Stewardship & Toxicology, Phillips 66, Bartlesville, OK 74003, USA; [b] Health Effects Laboratory Division, National Institute for Occupational Safety and Health, Morgantown, WV 26505, USA
* Corresponding author. National Institute for Occupational Safety and Health, 1095 Willowdale Drive, Morgantown, WV 26505.
*E-mail address:* sanderson4@cdc.gov

Immunol Allergy Clin N Am 41 (2021) 423–438
https://doi.org/10.1016/j.iac.2021.04.003
0889-8561/21/Published by Elsevier Inc.
immunology.theclinics.com

assay also uses a guinea pig model, where animals are dermally exposed to the test agent for 6 hours for 3 consecutive weeks. Two weeks after the final patch exposure, the animals are challenged by patch test of the flank for 6 hours[3] to measure the elicitation phase of allergy. Limitations of these assays include limited dose selection range (based on skin irritation threshold) and the use of single induction and challenge concentrations determined from range finding studies, which does not allow for dose response or evaluation of potency, but does provide valuable information for allergen identification.[4] In spite of these limitations, guinea pig-based sensitization assessment assays have significant utility, including a substantial test database, allowing for comparisons to new test agents and information regarding the elicitation phase of allergy.[4]

Currently, the gold standard for hazard identification of dermal sensitizers is the local lymph node assay (LLNA). This assay has been validated among independent laboratories,[5,6] with the United States-based Interagency Coordinating Committee on the Validation of Alternative Methods (ICCVAM)[7] and the European-based European Center for the Validation of Alternative Methods (ECVAM)[1] leading the validation exercises. The LLNA was adopted as TG 429 by the OECD in 2002.[8] The LLNA is based on the concept that repeated dermal exposure to sensitizers causes lymphocyte proliferation in draining lymph nodes (dLNs) proximal to the site of chemical application and that this proliferation can be quantified by using tritiated thymidine ($^3$H), which is incorporated into dLN DNA. **Fig. 1** illustrates the basic protocol of the LLNA. The assay uses female mice (preferably the CBA/Ca or CBA/J strain) at a minimum of 4 mice per group. A test substance is generally considered a sensitizer if it exhibits a dose-responsive increase in dLN proliferation from which the estimated concentration of test substance required to induce a stimulation index of at least 3 (EC3) can be determined. This value indicates a threefold or greater increase in dLN cell proliferation compared with vehicle-control mice. In general, predictive tests

## LLNA Overview

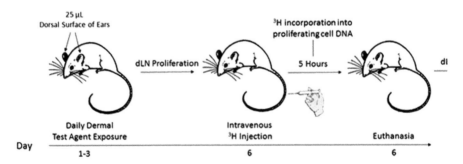

**Fig. 1.** Pictorial overview of the LLNA. Mice are dermally exposed on the dorsal surface of each ear to the vehicle, increasing concentrations of the test agent or a positive control for 3 consecutive days. After 3 days, mice are intravenously injected with $^3$H-thymidine ($^3$H) and euthanized 5 hours later; draining lymph nodes (dLNs) are excised and processed into single cell suspensions. These suspensions are tested for $^3$H incorporation based on disintegration per minute (DPM) readings. Results are expressed as the stimulation index (SI), which is the ratio of dLN allergen treated/control $^3$H incorporation.

exhibit certain limitations and results must be interpreted accordingly. The LLNA is not effective in identifying nickel salts (presumably because of variation in TLR4 signaling between mice and people); it exhibits false positives (specifically regarding nonsensitizing irritants)[9,10] and cannot distinguish between dermal and respiratory sensitizers. Regardless, the LLNA exhibits many advantages over other animal-based sensitization assays, including quick turnover and cost-effectiveness, less animal trauma, an end point directly associated with sensitization, dose response analysis yielding an index of potency (EC3 value), and close correlation between EC3 and human skin sensitization data.[4] There are also 2 nonradioactive modifications to the LLNA, the LLNA: DA (OECD TG 442A)[11] and LLNA: BrdU-ELISA (OECD TG 442B),[12] which assess the lymphocyte proliferation using nonradioactive methods.

### In Chemico, In Vitro, and In Silico Tests

Recently, experimental focus has been on the development of nonanimal alternatives to the LLNA and guinea pig methods. The major challenge in the development of in silico, in chemico, and in vitro alternatives for hazard identification of skin sensitizers is the ability to recapitulate the complex in vivo environment of an organism undergoing sensitization. The key chemical and biological events underlying skin sensitization and ACD, which have been extensively studied and are now generally understood,[9,13–16] were harnessed to establish an adverse outcome pathway (AOP) for skin sensitization[17,18] (**Fig. 2**). The mechanistic knowledge of key events (KEs) within the AOP framework enabled the development, validation, and acceptance of in chemico and in vitro methods for hazard identification of skin sensitizers. The clinical manifestation of ACD requires several steps to occur before the involvement of cell types including keratinocytes, Langerhans cells, dendritic cells, and T-lymphocytes.[19] The OECD adopted and developed the AOP framework,[17,18] which is defined as a chain of sequential causally related KEs, starting from a molecular initiating event (MIE) and ending in an adverse outcome (AO).[20] The in chemico and in vitro assays are based on one of the 4 AOP KEs, as illustrated in **Fig. 2**. It is worth noting that physicochemical properties of contact allergens (eg, chemical structure, molecular weight, physical state, pKa, Log Kow, vapor pressure, and water solubility) included in the AOP are important. Skin surface oxidation (for prehaptens), dermal penetration, skin metabolism (for prohaptens), and protein reactivity depend on these properties.

**Table 1** lists the currently available, validated in chemico and in vitro test methods.[21–29] Assays with designated OECD TG went through extensive evaluation and validation exercises conducted by national and international agencies such as ICCVAM, ECVAM, and Japanese Center for the Validation of Alternative Methods (JACVAM) to gauge their performance before OECD adoption. These OECD TGs are not considered stand-alone replacements for the animal tests given the multiple steps and complexity described in the AOP for skin sensitization. The assays need to be combined to be able to encompass the whole AOP framework. As such, an

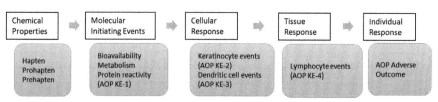

**Fig. 2.** Skin sensitization AOP and validated KEs within the AOP. The AOP was central to the development of in chemico and in vitro tests for low molecular weight (<1 kDa) chemicals.

**Table 1**
**In chemico and in vitro test methods for skin sensitization**

| Adverse Outcome Pathway Phase | In Chemico/Vitro Test Methods | Description |
|---|---|---|
| Dermal bioavailability | OECD TG 428[21] (skin absorption) | Skin permeation model representing the stratum corneum and viable skin (epidermis and dermis) where a test substance is applied to the surface of a skin sample separating the 2 chambers of a diffusion cell; the receptor fluid is sampled at intervals and analyzed for the test chemical and/or metabolites to measure the skin permeation |
| AOP KE-1: protein haptenation | OECD TG 442C[22] (DPRA) | In chemico test: quantification of the reactivity of test chemicals toward model synthetic peptides containing either lysine or cysteine; cysteine and lysine percent peptide depletion values are used in a prediction model to categorize a substance in 1 of 4 classes of peptide reactivity for supporting the discrimination between skin sensitizers and nonsensitizers |
| AOP KE-2: keratinocyte responses | Activation of biochemical pathways | |
| | OECD TG 442D[23] (ARE-Nrf2 luciferase test method)<br>1. KeratinoSens[23]<br>2. LuSens[23–25] | Perturbation of a cell line containing the luciferase gene under the transcriptional control of a constitutive promoter fused with an antioxidant/electrophile response element (ARE) element from a gene that is known to be up-regulated by contact sensitizers allows quantitative measurement (by luminescence detection) of luciferase gene induction as an indicator of the activity of the Nrf2 transcription factor in cells following exposure to electrophilic test substances; currently, 2 in vitro test methods are covered by this TG: the KeratinoSens assay and the LuSens assay |

(continued on next page)

| Table 1 (continued) | | |
|---|---|---|
| **Adverse Outcome Pathway Phase** | **In Chemico/Vitro Test Methods** | **Description** |
| AOP KE-3: dendritic cell responses | Expression of costimulatory and adhesion molecules in dendritic/monocytic cells OECD TG 442E[26] 1. Human cell line activation test (h-CLAT)[26] 2. U937 cell line activation test (U-SENS)[26,27] 3. Interleukin-8 (IL-8) reporter gene assay[26,28] | TG covers all 3 tests that are used to support the discrimination between skin sensitizers and nonsensitizers; change in the expression of cell surface marker(s) associated with the process of activation of monocytes and DC following exposure to sensitizers (eg, CD54, CD86) or changes in IL-8 expression, a cytokine associated with the activation of DC, is quantified in these assays; relative fluorescence or luminescence intensity of the treated cells versus controls is calculated and used to support the discrimination between sensitizers and nonsensitizers |
| AOP KE-4: tissue response | 1. The lymphocyte *ex-vivo* transformation test (LTT)[29] | The basis is that exposure in culture of primed memory T-lymphocytes to the relevant antigen will trigger a secondary response that reflects the acquisition of skin sensitization |
| AOP adverse outcome | — | — |

integrated approach to testing and assessment (IATA) is recommended if a decision on whether a test chemical is a sensitizer is to be made based on in vitro testing alone.[30] Combining tests such as the Direct Peptide Reactivity Assay (DPRA, KE-1), KeratinoSens assay (KE-2) and the Human Cell Line Activation Test (h- CLAT, KE-3) leads to test results that are acceptable. IATAs using combinations of these assays have been evaluated for regulatory application, some of which outperform animal tests to predict human skin sensitization.[30–35] It is important to point out that performing these assays requires the use of competent laboratories and scientists. In silico methods focused on predicting chemical reactivity based on the known in vivo reactivity of chemicals bearing structural significance are known as quantitative structural activity relationship (QSARs). There are also numerous in silico expert systems available such as the TImes MEtabolism Simulator platform (TIMES-SS) and Meteor Nexus that are simulators for skin metabolism, autoxidation, and reactivity. Some of these are available within the OECD QSAR Toolbox.[36]

### Current Regulatory Agency-Accepted Test Methods

Regulatory agencies in the United States and other developed countries have been increasing their general acceptance of the use of in vitro methods to obtain skin sensitization data to support decision making such as chemical registrations.[37] These agencies include the US Environmental Protection Agency (EPA), US Food and Drug Administration (FDA), Consumer Product Safety Commission (CPSC),

Occupational Safety and Health Administration (OSHA), European Chemicals Agency (ECHA), and the European Commission (EU) Cosmetics Regulation (EC) No. 1223/2009. Although all these agencies, except the European Commission, still require animal testing data for product safety evaluations and approvals, the agencies acknowledge the widely accepted AOP for skin sensitization and as such accept submission of in vitro testing data to support weight of evidence (WoE) evaluations.[37,38] In 2013, the Cosmetics Regulation (EC No. 1223/2009) banned animal use in cosmetics testing,[38,39] hence all testing for skin sensitization is now being performed using nonanimal methods such as the OECD TGs described.

## QUALITY CONTROL FOR PATCH TEST ALLERGENS, ALLERGEN STABILITY DATA

At present, the only FDA-approved percutaneous patch test system available is the T.R.U.E TEST. This test consists of 3 different allergen panels comprising a total of 35 allergen and allergen mixes along with a vehicle control contained in the ready-to-use panels. Most patch test allergens and allergen mixes that are not FDA approved are in a petrolatum or water vehicle and supplied in a syringe or dropper bottle. For these preparations, multiple allergens are added to patch test chambers to create patch test panels for diagnostic ACD testing.

Independent of the type of patch test, stability of allergen preparations is critical to prevent false-negative results and irritant reactions caused by product breakdown. Multiple studies pointing to storage instability of specific patch test allergen preparations were previously reviewed by Joy and colleagues[40] and Jou and colleagues[41] Loss of some allergens upon storage or preloading of patch test chambers has been demonstrated qualitatively/semiquantitatively, and/or quantitatively. The qualitative/semiquantitative studies were those that evaluated change of allergic subject patch test reactivity between fresh and stored preparations, while the quantitative test of contact allergen patch test reagents requires complex analytical laboratory analyses. **Table 2** provides a list of allergen stability laboratory studies reviewed by Jou and colleagues[41] along with the patch test allergen matrix and specific findings. Often it can be a challenge to extract the allergen from petrolatum into a solvent suitable for analysis, and extraction protocols can vary considerably depending on the chemical nature of the allergen(s) and the patch test vehicle. It is critical for the analytical laboratory to establish a standard with a known amount of allergen distributed uniformly in petrolatum to develop an extraction method that optimizes allergen recovery. Following development and validation of extraction protocols, quantitation of the allergens within a patch test preparation may be as simple as using a spectrophotometric chemical assay or as complex as requiring the use of chromatographic-mass spectrometric instrumentation.

Issues with allergen stability may be caused by physical and chemical properties of the chemical contact allergen. It has been documented that an allergen's high vapor pressure (volatility) can contribute to loss of the allergen from a patch test reagent, and particularly once the reagent is dispensed into a patch chamber.[42–44] Jou and colleagues[41] recommended that volatile allergens, such as formaldehyde, methyl methacrylate, and fragrances, be stored at lower temperatures in air-tight multidose containers, or sealed single-application containers, and aliquoted and prepared immediately before application. These recommendations would also decrease loss of allergens that are subject to air oxidation. Other possible causes of allergen loss with storage may be from self-polymerization, absorption or reaction with storage container surfaces, and reaction with other chemicals in the preparation. Additionally, loss of allergen may occur during compounding because of volatility[45] or possibly

**Table 2**
Patch test allergen stability

| Allergen/Vehicle | Instrumentation/Method | Finding | Reference |
|---|---|---|---|
| Thiuram mix/PET: tetramethylthiuram monosulfide (TMTM), tetramethylthiuram disulfide (TMTD), tetraethylthiuram disulfide (TETD) and dipentamethylenethiuram disulfide (PTD) | HPLC-UV/VIS | Thiuram mixes were unstable with individual thiurams reacting with each other to form mixed disulfides | Bergendorff & Hansson,[66] 2001 |
| Balsam of Peru/PET<br>Cobalt chloride/PET<br>Colophony/PET<br>Ethylenediamine/PET<br>Mercaptobenzothiazole/PET<br>Nickel sulfate/PET<br>Potassium dichromate/PET<br>Vioform/PET<br>Disperse yellow 3/PET<br>Formaldehyde/water | TLC or colorimetry | All found to be stable for 6 y in original sealed packaging, at room temperature, except formaldehyde, which had lower than acceptable levels in new and stored samples | Lembo et al,[67] 1993 |
| Methyldibromo glutaronitrile/PET | HPLC-UV | Stable for 1 y of storage at 6–8°C | Gruvberger et al,[68] 2004 |
| Cinnamal<br>Eugenol<br>Methyl methacrylate (MMA)<br>2-hydroxyethyl methacrylate (2-HEMA)<br>2-hydroxypropylacrylate | HPLC-diode array detector and GC-MS | All except 2-HEMA unstable if stored in patch test chambers at both 4°C and 22°C; all were more stable stored in a Vander Bend transport container | Mose et al,[44] 2012 |
| Tixocortol, pivalate, budesonide and hydrocortisone-17-butyrate (Hc-17-B)/pet, or ethanolic solution, or ethanol | HPLC-UV | All stable over a 50-week period except 1% Hc-17-B in ethanol | Isaksson et al,[69] 2000 |
| MMA<br>2-hydroxyethyl methacrylate<br>2-hydroxypropylacrylate (2-HPA)<br>ethylene glycoldimethacrylate<br>triethyleneglycoldiacrylate | HPLC-MS | 2-HPA and MMA predominately had unacceptable levels (<20% of the labeled concentration within the expiration date) | Goon et al,[46] 2011 |

*(continued on next page)*

**Table 2**
*(continued)*

| Allergen/Vehicle | Instrumentation/Method | Finding | Reference |
|---|---|---|---|
| Nickel sulfate/PET<br>Methyl methacrylate/PET<br>Formaldehyde/water<br>Glutaraldehyde/PET | Spectrophotometric measurement<br>GC-MS<br>Spectrophotometric measurement<br>Spectrophotometric measurement | Nickel and formaldehyde were at or above labeled patch test concentrations, but formaldehyde loss occurred with storage; lower than labeled concentrations of methyl methacrylate and glutaraldehyde concentrations were found in commercial patch test preparations independent of expiration date | Siegel et al,[45] 2014 |
| D-Limonene oxidation products/PET | HPLC-UV and GC-MS | Stable for 6 weeks when stored at 6–8°C Unstable if PET is stabilized with α-tocopheryl acetate | Nilsson et al,[70] 1999 |
| Fragrance mix 1/PET components – amyl cinnamal, cinnamal, cinnamyl alcohol, eugenol, geraniol, hydroxycitronella isoeugenol; E prunastri extract/PET-sorbitan sesquiol | HPLC-diode array detector or gel permeation chromatography-diode array detector[1] | At 23°C rapid time-dependent losses were observed for all fragrances in the mix or individually stored in Finn or IQ chambers Storage at 5°C slowed down the losses | Mowitz et al,[42] 2012 |
| Lyral/Pet | Gel permeation chromatography-UV detector | Losses observed when stored in Finn or IQ chambers above 5°C at 8 h; minimal loss after 9 d at 5°C | Hamann et al,[43] 2013 |
| Triglycidyl isocyanurate (TI) powder TI/PET | HPLC-UV detector | Degradation of TI observed in both powder and TI/PET in samples stored, refrigerated for 8 y | Erikstam et al,[71] 2015 |
| 2,4-Toluene diisocyanate (TDI)/PET<br>1,6-hexamethylene diisocyanate (HDI)/PET<br>Isophorone diisocyanate (IPDI)/PET | HPLC-MS | TDI, HDI and IPDI were all found to be stable and at the stated concentration in commercial preparations | Frick-Engfeldt et al,[72] 2005 |

| | HPLC-MS | diphenylmethane-4,4'-diisocyanate(MDI))/PET | MDI concentrations were lower than the labeled amount in commercial patch test preparations | Frick et al,[73] 2005 |
| | HPLC-MS | MDI, and polymeric (pMDI))/PET | Time and temperature dependent instability of both MDI. pMDI loss also observed except when stored in he freezer | Frick-Engfeldt et al,[74] 2007 |

because of compounding errors.[46] Because petrolatum is a solid at room temperature with a melting point of 70 to 80°C, the compounding process may require melting petrolatum or extensive mixing to obtain a uniform distribution of the allergen.

## CHEMISTRY LABORATORY DERMATOLOGIST SUPPORT

The potential role of laboratory chemistry in clinical ACD diagnosis includes confirmation of etiologic allergens in patients' products, unknown allergen identification, and development and evaluation of allergen spot tests. These activities differ from the traditional clinical laboratory testing, and impediments exist in implementation of chemical laboratory analyses for individual patient diagnosis and counseling. De Groot[47] surveyed the journals, Contact Dermatitis and Dermatitis, between 2008 and 2015, and found 172 new contact allergens that were identified by patch testing. This is likely an underestimate of new contact allergen exposures, as not all cases are reported in the literature, patch testing of potential causative materials is often not performed, and the specific etiologic chemical agent goes unidentified. At present, identification and possible quantification of allergens from products associated with ACD have been mostly limited to research studies and case reports of new, novel allergens because of the complexity and cost of such chemical analyses.

Dermatologists identify contact allergens to which their patients react through clinical history and the use of dermal patch testing. They can verify if a product (eg, personal care products or clothing) used by the patient is associated with the patient's allergy through product patch testing. However, it can be more problematic confirming the presence of the patch test-positive allergen in the suspect material. Siegel and colleagues[48] found that the patient's ability to identify the glove source of their ACD was directly related to the severity of their patch test reaction to the rubber allergen, and inversely related to the number of different rubber glove types in use by the patient. It was concluded that in the absence of chemical analysis of a patient's possible ACD-causative gloves, all of the patient's rubber gloves need to be considered as potential sources of the contact allergen.

Product content labels or even safety data sheets (SDSs) are not always reliable for allergen identification. Multiple studies have demonstrated the presence of undeclared allergens or absence of declared allergens by product chemical analyses for the suspect allergens. For example, undeclared isothiazolinones have been documented in several reports of products such as gel face mask,[49] emulsifying oil,[50] wall paints,[51,52] and dish soap[53]; undeclared dehydroabietic acid in neoprene surgical gloves[54]; and undeclared formaldehyde/formaldehyde releaser in personal products,[55–57] baby wipes,[58] and tattoo ink.[59] The presence of these undeclared contact allergens may be due to several reasons including presence in the raw materials used in the product production, mislabeling, or contamination from machinery treated with biocides.[53]

Reliable labeling and SDSs would be the most expedient and cost-effective tool to confirm allergen clinical relevance of a patient's patch test result. However, a manufacturer may consider an ingredient as proprietary and be reluctant to provide more specific product content or confirm the presence of a specific chemical. In such cases, chemical analysis to assess if the material contains a suspect allergen(s) would provide strong evidence of clinical relevance to the allergen patch test results; however, obstacles to widespread contact allergen product testing exist. Methodological considerations for confirmation of etiologic allergen content of patient products and identification of unknown allergens was recently reviewed by Siegel and colleagues,[60] as well as by Gruberger and colleagues[61] Although confirmation of the presence of a specific contact allergen(s) in a suspect material does not need to involve a quantitative analysis, the extraction and measurement procedures should be sufficiently robust to avoid false-negative or false-positive analytical results. The product matrices can also vary substantially from product to product, which may require substantial method modifications to extract the contact allergen from the product into a solvent that is compatible with the analytical chemical detection method. Chemical detection methods can range from a simple spot test to highly sophisticated chromatographic mass spectrometric analyses. The more sophisticated instrumentation may add a greater level of confidence in the allergen identification confirmation, but this can also significantly increase the cost of the analysis. If quantitative analysis of the amount of the allergen in the product is desired, additional steps would be required to evaluate the extraction recovery and the precision and accuracy of the measurement method.

9Spot tests are simple qualitative or semiquantitative tests that use small amounts of sample, reagents, and test steps to yield fast results that usually consist of a color change. There are commercially available spot test kits for only a few chemical allergens, and most have not been validated for the various matrices/products associated with ACD reactions. The authors have recently reported on the utility of various kits for detection of formaldehyde[56] and isothiazolinones[53] marketed for water analyses. The chemical detection-based formaldehyde test strip kits were found to have utility in detecting formaldehyde from the consumer products tested, while the enzyme-based kit was unreliable. The accuracy of the isothiazolinone test kit was very poor for detection of isothiazolinones in dish soaps and personal care products. Test kits are also available for several metals including nickel, cobalt, and hexavalent chromium.

Identification of an unknown contact allergen in the absence of an a priori postulated chemical structure can be complex and costly. Bruze and colleagues[62] developed a thin layer chromatographic patch test that can aid in separation of a product's chemical components and segregation of the contact allergens. If the contact allergen is compatible with gas chromatographic-electron impact-mass spectral analyses (GC-EI-MS) and the resultant electron impact ion spectra matches that from an MS library, a tentative chemical identification can be made. Chemical identity should be confirmed against a chemical standard when one is available. Many chemical contact allergens cannot be assayed directly using GC-EI-MS or have a spectrum that is not in an MS library. For these instances, further analyses using ultrahigh performance liquid chromatography with tandem mass spectrometry (UHPLC-MS-MS) can be used to obtain the chemical's mass, isotopic distribution, and daughter ion fragments to determine a potential molecular formula. Two-dimensional proton nuclear magnetic resonance could be conducted; however, this technique requires milligram quantities of a pure substance to tentatively identify the chemical structure. Confirmation of the tentatively identified chemical would be performed by demonstration of identical chromatographic retention times and mass spectral ion chromatographs to that of a pure chemical standard. Such analyses may be prohibitively expensive, labor intensive and require high levels of expertise for routine implementation in patient diagnosis and counseling.

Identification of unknown allergens has been reported for synthetic and natural extracts used in the fragrance industry. Chaintreau and colleagues[63] reported a GC-MS method for quantification of 24 fragrance contact allergens; however, there remains unidentified fragrance contact allergens especially in natural extract fragrances. Oak moss extract is one such natural extract that is used in perfumes. It is a complex chemical mixture of greater than 170 compounds[64] and a cause of ACD. Although most fragrances are amenable to GC-MS analyses, the number of chemical components in the extract can present a challenge in the identification of the allergenic components. This is common with all chemical substances of unknown or variable composition, complex reaction products and biological materials (UVCBs). Oak moss extract is regarded as a UVCB substance. Bernard and colleagues[65] fractionated and subfractionated oak moss extracted using gel permeation and silica gel column chromatography, respectively, with all fractions testing positive in oak moss-allergic subjects. GC-MS analyses identified multiple potential allergens, but only a standard of chloroatranol/atranol elicited positive patch test reactions. This study demonstrates the complexity of identification of unknown specific chemical allergens from complex mixtures.

## CLINICS CARE POINTS

- Laboratory-based analyses are available to identify the skin sensitization hazard of potential chemical allergens.
- Commercially available patch test reagent storage instability may be a potential cause of a false-negative finding. Storage of volatile and labile reagents at lower temperatures can decrease allergen loss from patch test reagents.
- Few reliable chemical spot tests are available to clinicians to confirm that a patch test-positive chemical is in the product eliciting the allergic contact dermatitis. Laboratory-based chemical allergen identification can be complex and is generally unavailable for patient care.

## CONFLICT OF INTEREST

The authors declare no conflicts of interest. The authors alone are responsible for the content of this article. The findings and conclusions in this report are those of the authors and do not necessarily represent the official position of the National Institute for Occupational Safety and Health or the Centers for Disease Control and Prevention.

## REFERENCES

1. Anderson SE, Siegel PD, Meade BJ. The LLNA: a brief review of recent advances and limitations. J Allergy (Cairo) 2011;2011:424203.
2. OECD. Test No. 406: Skin Sensitisation, OECD guidelines for the testing of chemicals, Section 4. 1992. Paris. https://doi.org/10.1787/9789264070660-en.
3. Frankild S, Volund A, Wahlberg JE, et al. Comparison of the sensitivities of the Buehler test and the guinea pig maximization test for predictive testing of contact allergy. Acta Derm Venereol 2000;80(4):256–62.
4. Kimber I, Basketter DA, Berthold K, et al. Skin sensitization testing in potency and risk assessment. Toxicol Sci 2001;59(2):198–208.
5. Kimber I, Hilton J, Dearman RJ, et al. Assessment of the skin sensitization potential of topical medicaments using the local lymph node assay: an interlaboratory evaluation. J Toxicol Environ Health A 1998;53(7):563–79.
6. Loveless SE, Ladics GS, Gerberick GF, et al. Further evaluation of the local lymph node assay in the final phase of an international collaborative trial. Toxicology 1996;108(1–2):141–52.
7. Dean JH, Twerdok LE, Tice RR, et al. ICCVAM evaluation of the murine local lymph node assay. Conclusions and recommendations of an independent scientific peer review panel. Regul Toxicol Pharmacol 2001;34(3):258–73.

8.  OECD. Test No. 429: Skin Sensitisation: Local Lymph Node Assay, OECD guidelines for the testing of chemicals, Section 4. 2010. Paris. https://doi.org/10.1787/9789264071100-en.

9.  Kimber I, Basketter DA, Gerberick GF, et al. Chemical allergy: translating biology into hazard characterization. Toxicol Sci 2011;120(Suppl 1):S238–68.

10. Montelius J, Wahlkvist H, Boman A, et al. Murine local lymph node assay for predictive testing of allergenicity: two irritants caused significant proliferation. Acta Derm Venereol 1998;78(6):433–7.

11. OECD. Test No. 442A: skin sensitization: local lymph node assay: DA, OECD, guidelines for the testing of chemicals, Section 4. 2010. OECD Publishing, Paris. https://doi.org/10.1787/9789264090972-en.

12. OECD. Test No. 442B: skin sensitization: local lymph node assay: BrdU-ELISA or–FCM, OECD guidelines for the testing of chemicals, Section 4. 2018. Paris, OECD Publishing.

13. Adler S, Basketter D, Creton S, et al. Alternative (non-animal) methods for cosmetics testing: current status and future prospects-2010. Arch Toxicol 2011; 85(5):367–485.

14. Karlberg AT, Bergstrom MA, Borje A, et al. Allergic contact dermatitis–formation, structural requirements, and reactivity of skin sensitizers. Chem Res Toxicol 2008; 21(1):53–69.

15. Martin SF, Esser PR, Schmucker S, et al. T-cell recognition of chemicals, protein allergens and drugs: towards the development of in vitro assays. Cell Mol Life Sci 2010;67(24):4171–84.

16. Vocanson M, Hennino A, Rozieres A, et al. Effector and regulatory mechanisms in allergic contact dermatitis. Allergy 2009;64(12):1699–714.

17. OECD. The adverse outcome pathway for skin sensitisation initiated by covalent binding to Proteins, OECD Series on Testing and Assessment, No. 168, 2014. OECD Publishing, Paris, https://doi.org/10.1787/9789264221444-en.

18. OECD. The adverse outcome pathway for skin sensitisation initiated by covalent binding to proteins. Part 2: use of the AOP to develop chemical categories and integrated assessment and testing approaches. Series on testing and assessment No. 168;ENV/JM/MONO(2012)10/PART2 2012. Available at: https://www.oecd.org/officialdocuments/publicdisplaydocumentpdf/?cote=env/jm/mono%282012%2910/part2&doclanguage=en.

19. de Avila RI, Lindstedt M, Valadares MC. The 21st century movement within the area of skin sensitization assessment: From the animal context towards current human-relevant in vitro solutions. Regul Toxicol Pharmacol 2019;108:104445.

20. FitzGerald RE. Adverse outcome pathway bridge building from research to regulation. Chem Res Toxicol 2020;33(4):849–51.

21. OECD. Test No. 428: skin absorption: in vitro method, OECD guidelines for the testing of chemicals, Section 4, OECD Publishing, Paris, https://doi.org/10.1787/9789264071087-en.

22. OECD. Test No. 442C: In Chemico Skin Sensitisation: Assays addressing the Adverse Outcome Pathway key event on covalent binding to proteins, OECD Guidelines for the Testing of Chemicals, Section 4, 2020. OECD Publishing, Paris, https://doi.org/10.1787/9789264229709-en.

23. OECD. Test No. 442D: in vitro skin sensitisation: ARE-Nrf2 luciferase test Method, OECD guidelines for the testing of chemicals, Section 4. 2018. Paris. https://doi.org/10.1787/9789264229822-en.

24. Ramirez T, Mehling A, Kolle SN, et al. LuSens: a keratinocyte based ARE reporter gene assay for use in integrated testing strategies for skin sensitization hazard identification. Toxicol In Vitro 2014;28(8):1482–97.

25. Ramirez T, Stein N, Aumann A, et al. Intra- and inter-laboratory reproducibility and accuracy of the LuSens assay: a reporter gene-cell line to detect keratinocyte activation by skin sensitizers. Toxicol In Vitro 2016;32:278–86.

26. OECD. Test No. 442E: In vitro skin Sensitisation: In vitro skin sensitisation assays addressing the key event on activation of dendritic cells on the adverse outcome pathway for skin Sensitisation, OECD guidelines for the testing of chemicals, Section 4. 2018. OECD Publishing, Paris. https://doi.org/10.1787/9789264264359-en.

27. Piroird C, Ovigne JM, Rousset F, et al. The Myeloid U937 Skin Sensitization Test (U-SENS) addresses the activation of dendritic cell event in the adverse outcome pathway for skin sensitization. Toxicol In Vitro 2015;29(5):901–16.

28. Kimura Y, Fujimura C, Ito Y, et al. Optimization of the IL-8 Luc assay as an in vitro test for skin sensitization. Toxicol In Vitro 2015;29(7):1816–30.

29. Popple A, Williams J, Maxwell G, et al. The lymphocyte transformation test in allergic contact dermatitis: new opportunities. J Immunotoxicol 2016;13(1):84–91.

30. Patlewicz G, Kuseva C, Kesova A, et al. Towards AOP application–implementation of an integrated approach to testing and assessment (IATA) into a pipeline tool for skin sensitization. Regul Toxicol Pharmacol 2014;69(3):529–45.

31. Kimura Y, Watanabe M, Suzuki N, et al. The performance of an in vitro skin sensitisation test, IL-8 Luc assay (OECD442E), and the integrated approach with direct peptide reactive assay (DPRA). J Toxicol Sci 2018;43(12):741–9.

32. Kleinstreuer NC, Hoffmann S, Alepee N, et al. Non-animal methods to predict skin sensitization (II): an assessment of defined approaches (*). Crit Rev Toxicol 2018; 48(5):359–74.

33. Natsch A, Ryan CA, Foertsch L, et al. A dataset on 145 chemicals tested in alternative assays for skin sensitization undergoing prevalidation. J Appl Toxicol 2013; 33(11):1337–52.

34. OECD, Guidance. Document on the reporting of defined approaches to be used within integrated approaches to testing and assessment Series on testing and assessment No. 256. Paris: OECD Publishing; 2016.

35. Strickland J, Zang Q, Kleinstreuer N, et al. Integrated decision strategies for skin sensitization hazard. J Appl Toxicol 2016;36(9):1150–62.

36. OECD. The OECD QSAR toolbox 2014. Available at: https://www.oecd.org/chemicalsafety/risk-assessment/oecd-qsar-toolbox.htm.

37. Strickland J, Daniel AB, Allen D, et al. Skin sensitization testing needs and data uses by US regulatory and research agencies. Arch Toxicol 2019;93(2):273–91.

38. Daniel AB, Strickland J, Allen D, et al. International regulatory requirements for skin sensitization testing. Regul Toxicol Pharmacol : RTP 2018;95:52–65.

39. EU. Regulation (EC) No 1223/2009 Of the European parliament and of the council of 30 November 2009 on cosmetic products 2009. Available at: https://www.legislation.gov.uk/eur/2009/1223/contents.

40. Joy NM, Rice KR, Atwater AR. Stability of patch test allergens. Dermatitis 2013; 24(5):227–36.

41. Jou PC, Siegel PD, Warshaw EM. Vapor pressure and predicted stability of American contact dermatitis society core allergens. Dermatitis 2016;27(4):193–201.

42. Mowitz M, Zimerson E, Svedman C, et al. Stability of fragrance patch test preparations applied in test chambers. Br J Dermatol 2012;167(4):822–7.

43. Hamann D, Hamann CR, Zimerson E, et al. Hydroxyisohexyl 3-cyclohexene car-boxaldehyde (lyral) in patch test preparations under varied storage conditions. Dermatitis 2013;24(5):246–8.
44. Mose KF, Andersen KE, Christensen LP. Stability of selected volatile contact aller-gens in different patch test chambers under different storage conditions. Contact Dermatitis 2012;66(4):172–9.
45. Siegel PD, Fowler JF, Law BF, et al. Concentrations and stability of methyl meth-acrylate, glutaraldehyde, formaldehyde and nickel sulfate in commercial patch test allergen preparations. Contact Dermatitis 2014;70(5):309–15.
46. Goon AT, Bruze M, Zimerson E, et al. Correlation between stated and measured concentrations of acrylate and methacrylate allergens in patch-test preparations. Dermatitis 2011;22(1):27–32.
47. de Groot AC. New contact allergens: 2008 to 2015. Dermatitis 2015;26(5): 199–215.
48. Siegel PD, Fowler JF Jr, Storrs FJ, et al. Allergen content of patient problem and nonproblem gloves: relationship to allergen-specific patch-test findings. Derma-titis 2010;21(2):77–83.
49. Kerre S, Naessens T, Theunis M, et al. Facial dermatitis caused by undeclared methylisothiazolinone in a gel mask: is the preservation of raw materials in cos-metics a cause of concern? Contact Dermatitis 2018;78(6):421–4.
50. Corazza M, Forconi R, Bernardi T, et al. Occupational allergic contact dermatitis due to undeclared benzisothiazolinone in an emulsifying oil. Contact Dermatitis 2020;83(5):408–9.
51. Aerts O, Meert H, Goossens A, et al. Methylisothiazolinone in selected consumer products in Belgium: adding fuel to the fire? Contact Dermatitis 2015;73(3): 142–9.
52. Goodier MC, Siegel PD, Zang LY, et al. Isothiazolinone in residential interior wall paint: a high-performance liquid chromatographic-mass spectrometry analysis. Dermatitis 2018;29(6):332–8.
53. Kimyon RS, Siegel PD, Voller LM, et al. Isothiazolinone detection in dish soap and personal care products: comparison of Lovibond isothiazolinone test kit and ultra high performance liquid chromatographic tandem mass spectrometry. Dermatitis 2020. in press.
54. Siegel PD, Law BF, Fowler JF Jr, et al. Disproportionated rosin dehydroabietic acid in neoprene surgical gloves. Dermatitis 2010;21(3):157–9.
55. Nikle A, Ericson M, Warshaw E. Formaldehyde release from personal care prod-ucts: chromotropic acid method analysis. Dermatitis 2019;30(1):67–73.
56. Ham JE, Siegel PD, Maibach H. Undeclared formaldehyde levels in patient con-sumer products: formaldehyde test kit utility. Cutan Ocul Toxicol 2019;38(2): 112–7.
57. Gruvberger B, Bruze M, Tammela M. Preservatives in moisturizers on the Swedish market. Acta Derm Venereol 1998;78(1):52–6.
58. Liou YL, Ericson ME, Warshaw EM. Formaldehyde release from baby wipes: anal-ysis using the chromotropic acid method. Dermatitis 2019;30(3):207–12.
59. Liou YL, Voller LM, Liszewski W, et al. Formaldehyde Release From Predispersed Tattoo Inks: Analysis Using the Chromotropic Acid Method. Dermatitis. 2020.
60. Siegel PD, Law BF, Warshaw EM. Chemical identification and confirmation of con-tact allergens. Dermatitis 2020;31(2):99–105.
61. Gruvberger B, Bruze M, Fregert S. Spot tests and chemical analyses for allergen evaluation. In: Rycroft RJG, Menné T, Frosch PJ, et al, editors. Textbook of con-tact dermatitis. Berlin, Heidelberg: Springer Berlin Heidelberg; 2001. p. 495–510.

62. Bruze M, Frick M, Persson L. Patch testing with thin-layer chromatograms. Contact Dermatitis 2003;48(5):278–9.

63. Chaintreau A, Joulain D, Marin C, et al. GC-MS quantitation of fragrance compounds suspected to cause skin reactions. 1. J Agric Food Chem 2003;51(22): 6398–403.

64. Mowitz M, Zimerson E, Svedman C, et al. Patch testing with serial dilutions and thin-layer chromatograms of oak moss absolutes containing high and low levels of atranol and chloroatranol. Contact Dermatitis 2013;69(6):342–9.

65. Bernard G, Giménez-Arnau E, Rastogi SC, et al. Contact allergy to oak moss: search for sensitizing molecules using combined bioassay-guided chemical fractionation, GC-MS, and structure-activity relationship analysis. Arch Dermatol Res 2003;295(6):229–35.

66. Bergendorff O, Hansson C. Stability of thiuram disulfides in patch test preparations and formation of asymmetric disulfides. Contact Dermatitis 2001;45(3): 151–7.

67. Lembo G, Patruno C, Balato N, et al. Stability of patch test allergens. Contact Dermatitis 1993;29(2):95–6.

68. Gruvberger B, Bjerkemo M, Bruze M. Stability of patch test preparations of methyldibromo glutaronitrile in petrolatum. Contact Dermatitis 2004;51(5–6):315–6.

69. Isaksson M, Gruvberger B, Persson L, et al. Stability of corticosteroid patch test preparations. Contact Dermatitis 2000;42(3):144–8.

70. Nilsson U, Magnusson K, Karlberg O, et al. Are contact allergens stable in patch test preparations? Investigation of the degradation of d-limonene hydroperoxides in petrolatum. Contact Dermatitis 1999;40(3):127–32.

71. Erikstam U, Bruze M, Goossens A. Degradation of triglycidyl isocyanurate as a cause of false-negative patch test reaction. Contact Dermatitis 2001;44(1):13–7.

72. Frick-Engfeldt M, Zimerson E, Karlsson D, et al. Chemical analysis of 2,4-toluene diisocyanate, 1,6-hexamethylene diisocyanate and isophorone diisocyanate in petrolatum patch-test preparations. Dermatitis 2005;16(3):130–5.

73. Frick M, Zimerson E, Karlsson D, et al. Poor correlation between stated and found concentrations of diphenylmethane-4,4'-diisocyanate (4,4'-MDI) in petrolatum patch-test preparations. Contact Dermatitis 2004;51(2):73–8.

74. Frick-Engfeldt M, Isaksson M, Zimerson E, et al. How to optimize patch testing with diphenylmethane diisocyanate. Contact Dermatitis 2007;57(3):138–51.

# Occupational Dermatitis and Urticaria

Dorothy Linn Holness, MD, MHSc, DTS, FRCPC[a,b,c,]*

## KEYWORDS

- Occupational skin disease • Occupational contact dermatitis
- Occupational irritant contact dermatitis • Occupational allergic contact dermatitis
- Occupational contact urticaria • Prevention • Screening • Outcomes

## KEY POINTS

- Occupational skin disease (OSD) is common.
- OSD is preventable.
- Early detection of OSD leads to improved outcomes.
- Management includes both medical and workplace components.
- OSD has significant impact on a worker.

## INTRODUCTION

Occupational skin disease (OSD) is one of the most common occupational diseases. Contact dermatitis represents most of the cases. Contact dermatitis is an eczematous inflammatory skin reaction to direct contact with noxious agents in our environment, and in the case of occupational contact dermatitis (OCD) the agent is in the workplace.[1] Contact urticaria is a condition characterized by wheals and/or angioedema occurring after skin contact with a substance and for occupational contact urticaria (OCU), the substance is in the workplace.[2] Both may be the result of an allergic response to a workplace agent or a nonimmunologic response.

Occupational irritant contact dermatitis (OICD) accounts for approximately 80% of OCD. It is caused by contact with substances or mechanical stressors that have a direct toxic effect on the skin.[3] Some irritants may cause an acute OICD (chemical burn), whereas others are the result of exposure to irritants over a longer period of time. Occupational allergic contact dermatitis (OACD) occurs when a worker is sensitized via a delayed, type IV hypersensitivity reaction to a substance in the workplace.

[a] Department of Medicine and Dalla Lana School of Public Health, University of Toronto, Toronto, Ontario, Canada; [b] Division of Occupational Medicine, Department of Medicine, St Michael's Hospital, 30 Bond Street, Toronto, Ontario M5B 1W8, Canada; [c] MAP Centre for Urban Health Solutions, Li Ka Shing Knowledge Institute, St Michael's Hospital, 30 Bond Street, Toronto, Ontario M5B 1W8, Canada
* Department of Medicine and Dalla Lana School of Public Health, University of Toronto, Toronto, Ontario, Canada.
*E-mail address:* linn.holness@unityhealth.to

Immunol Allergy Clin N Am 41 (2021) 439–453
https://doi.org/10.1016/j.iac.2021.04.006
0889-8561/21/© 2021 Elsevier Inc. All rights reserved.
immunology.theclinics.com

OCU may be the result of an immune response to a workplace agent or a nonimmu-nologic response. It involves an immediate, type I hypersensitivity reaction.[3]

## EPIDEMIOLOGY
### Sources of Information

An important consideration in understanding the epidemiology of OSD, including the incidence and prevalence and also the causative agents and common industries and occupations associated with OSD, is understanding the sources of information and the strengths and limitations or each. We get an overall picture by considering all the sources of information and, if the findings are consistent across different types of sources, this increases our confidence in the information. Common limitations include underrecognition and underreporting of the work-related diseases and the ac-curacy of the diagnosis.

The main sources of information include (1) administrative data, (2) registries, (3) sur-veillance systems, (4) clinical databases, (5) workplace studies, and (6) case reports and case series. Following, the different methods will be reviewed, and information focused on findings in the health care sector will be used as examples of each.

### Administrative data—occupationally focused

There are several types of administrative data that are used: required government reporting and insurance schemes including workers' compensation. Burnett and col-leagues[4] reported on lost-time dermatitis cases from the Annual Survey of Occupa-tional Injuries and Illnesses from the Bureau of Labor statistics. They found an overall rate of 1.12 per 10,000 workers. Health services had the highest number of cases. Morse produced a comprehensive report for Connecticut that included infor-mation from the Bureau of Labor Statistics and their workers' compensation system.[5] Information from the Bureau of Labor Statistics from 2015 found 400 cases in a total of 302,015 cases. Education and health services had a rate of 3.1 per 10,000 workers. In the same report, Morse also reported on workers' compensation data and found 178 cases in the 2015 data. Gloves including latex were one of the key causes.

Specific issues can also be examined with workers' compensation data. Horwitz and colleagues[6] examined claims related to latex in Oregon health care workers from 1987 to 1998. They found an increase in claims related to latex over the time period. Dermatitis was the most common problem (80%), whereas 3% had urticaria. Malerich and colleagues[7] used workers' compensation data from 1997 to 2005 to demonstrate a decrease in latex-related claims following an intervention to eliminate powdered latex gloves from health care institutions in 2001. They found a decrease in claim incidence with an average incidence of 2.992 per 1000 at risk before the inter-vention to 0.92 per 1000 after the intervention.

### Registries

Some jurisdictions maintain registries of occupational disease. An example of a na-tional registry that recently reported its results from cases between 2005 and 2016 is the Finnish Register of Occupational Diseases.[8] The distribution of diagnoses for OICD, OACD, and OCU among all the OSD were 42%, 35%, and 11%, respectively. The incidence of OSD in the human health and social services sector was 25 per 100,000 persons. The main causes of OICD were wet work (35%), detergents (11%), dirty work (8%), and cutting fluids and oils (5%). The main causes of OACD were plastics and resins (29%), rubber/rubber chemicals (17%), preserva-tives (16%), epoxies (16%), and metals (12%). They also specifically examined the cases of OCU.[9] Most common occupations and their incidence per 10,000 were bakers, pastry cooks and confectionary makers (10.5), chefs (2.6), and cooks (1.8), respectively. The most common causes included animal dander and excretions (51%), flour, grain and animal feed (22%), and natural rubber latex (8.4%).

*Surveillance systems*
Another source of information is surveillance systems. As an example, there have been several occupational disease surveillance systems in the United Kingdom for several years. These include 2 reporting schemes that capture OSD. EPIDERM is a reporting system for dermatologists, and OPRA is a system for occupational physicians. A variety of information is generated from these surveillance schemes. McDonald and colleague[10] provided information on reported cases to the 2 schemes from 1996 to 2001, including information on incidence and occupation and industry. For the overall period 1996 to 2001, dermatologists reported an overall rate of OSD of 97 per million and occupational physicians a rate of 623 per million. OCD rates were 74 per million by dermatologists and 510 per million for occupational physicians, and the comparable rates for OCU were 4 and 31, respectively. The most common causative agents reported for OCD were rubber chemicals, soaps and cleaners, and wet work, and for OCU they were rubber chemicals and food and flours. In the Netherlands a similar scheme for dermatologist reporting found that of the total of 4516 cases reported between 2001 and 2005, 80% were OCD and 2% OCU.[11] Hairdressers and nurses were the 2 most common occupations represented, with 16% of the cases occurring in the health and welfare sector. The most common reported causative agents were irritants including wet work, irritating chemicals, and mechanical factors, and the most common allergens were hairdressing products, preservatives, rubber chemicals, plants, acrylates, and latex.

These surveillance systems can also be used to track changes over time. An example relates to latex allergy. Following the introduction of universal precautions, there was an epidemic of latex allergy in health care workers due to the use of latex gloves, particularly powdered gloves. Once latex was identified as a problem, latex gloves were replaced with other types of gloves such as nitrile of vinyl in many countries. Information from EPIDERM for the years 1996 to 2007 demonstrated not only the decrease in latex allergy following this change but also the increase in OICD related to an increase in handwashing after hand hygiene was emphasized after severe acute respiratory syndrome.[12]

Similarly, the decrease in latex as a causative agent was demonstrated in the Netherlands' scheme.[11] Another of the United Kingdom's reporting systems, THOR, was used to examine the changes that occurred with the increased focus on hand hygiene.[13] Examining the period from 1996 to 2012, they found that the incidence of irritant contact dermatitis in health care workers increased steadily, whereas the incidence in other workers declined. Bensefa-Colas and colleagues[14] reported on OCU from the French National Network for Occupational Disease Vigilance and Prevention for the period from 2001 to 2010. They found that half of latex-related OCU was in the health care and social work sectors, and they also documented the decrease in latex-related OCU over this time. Morse also reported on an occupational disease surveillance system in Connecticut.[5] In 2015, there were 116 dermatitis cases reported, with 42% being in the education and health care sector. Carder and colleagues[15] have provided a useful summary of occupational disease surveillance systems in European Union countries.

*Clinical sources*
A key source of information about causative allergens comes from clinic populations. Included are both reporting of clinical populations and also the results from patch test

databases containing patch test information. Clinicians pool their patch test results while using standardized protocols including sets of allergens and test methods. When these databases are continued over many years, not only can specific allergens be identified, but trends over time can also be observed. Two of the large clinical pooled patch test databases are the North American Contact Dermatitis Group (NACDG) and the European Surveillance System on Contact Allergy (ESSCA).[16,17] The NACDG reported occupational results in its 1998 to 2000 data. Of 369 cases of OSD, 46% were OICD, 33% OACD, and 4% OCU.[16] The most common occupational allergens were rubber chemicals (carba and thiuram), epoxy, formaldehyde, and nickel. Health care workplaces were the common source of exposure to the rubber components. The ESSCA reported its occupational data based on its 2002 to 2010 results.[17] The overall risk for OCD was 7.8 per 100,000 workers. In examining the health-related occupations, as examples, 39% of nurses had OICD, 29% had OACD, and 18% with both. In contrast, 47 of dental professionals had OACD and 23% had OICD and 11% with both. The most common occupational allergens were rubbers, epoxy resin, and preservatives. The routine use of standardized patch test haptens and the pooling of data have allowed for much more information related to OCD than with OCU.

In addition to patch test databases, there are also studies of clinic populations where there is more detailed reporting of their experience. An example is Higgins and colleagues[18] who describe health care workers seen in the Occupational Dermatology Clinic in Australia between 1993 and 2014. Of the 685 health care workers seen, 88% were diagnosed with OSD, including 79% with OICD and 50% with OACD. Natural rubber latex allergy was found in 13%. The common irritants were wet work and hand cleaners, and the common allergens were rubber glove chemicals and preservatives.

### Workplace studies

Workplace studies are another important source of information; however, there are relatively few, as they are more challenging to conduct and may be expensive to conduct. These include studies of workers in a particular workplace or workplaces. They also may not provide confirmed diagnostic information but usually provide information about symptoms and clinical findings. Health care is one of the sectors that has been studied at the workplace level.[19–22] These studies have reported a prevalence of hand dermatitis between 19% and 31%. These studies also provide information on risk factors. For hand dermatitis the key risk factors identified by the studies included a history of atopic dermatitis or history of atopy and hand washing.

In addition, some of these studies have a more detailed clinical assessment. For example, Ibler and colleagues[23] saw a subset of 120 health care workers of their study population who reported hand eczema. They were assessed with patch and prick testing. Of those assessed with patch testing, 53% had positive patch test reactions. The most common reactions were to nickel, thiomersal, fragrances, rubber chemicals, and colophony; however, an assessment of whether these positives were work related was not included. They also performed prick testing and specific immunoglobulin E (IgE) tests for natural rubber latex and chlorhexidine. Six workers had positive results for latex; however, only one was positive to both. One worker had a positive prick test to chlorhexidine.

### Case series and case reports

Although case series and case reports are not viewed as strong sources of evidence, they do play an important role in OSD in that new allergens are usually first described in case series or case reports. They are important sentinel cases to alert practitioners of potential new allergens or causative agents for both OCD and OCU and also new sources of exposure for known allergens. An example from the COVID-19 pandemic is the report by Aerts and colleagues[24] of OACD related to formaldehyde releasers in a surgical mask.

## PREVENTION

Having identified that OCD and OCU are common occupational diseases and also the key causative agents, a first question to be posed is how do we prevent OSD? A recent review of hand dermatitis in health care workers by Public Health Ontario addresses prevention.[25] The standard hierarchy of controls approach is used with the key interventions (in descending order of effectiveness) including elimination, substitution, engineering controls, administrative controls, and personal protective equipment.[25] Examples of these approaches in the case of health care workers would be the elimination of powdered latex gloves, the substitution of a harsh cleanser for one that contains emollients, providing needed cleansers and emollients at easily accessible locations, training related to preventing skin exposure and protecting the skin, and the use of gloves to protect the skin. Appropriate care of the skin is also important in the control of OSD.[25] In addition to the review focused on health care workers by Public Health Ontario and the review and recommendations for both OCD and OCU by Nicholson and colleagues, there have been several other reviews including a recent update of the Cochrane review of OICD.[3,26]

There is limited evidence about these interventions in working populations. One of the most studied and reported is the elimination of powdered latex gloves in health care institutions. As discussed earlier, there is clear evidence that the elimination resulted in decreased cases of latex allergy.

There are several interventions using a variety of prevention strategies in groups of workers that commonly experience OCD including health care workers. The interventions are usually training and the provision of hand hygiene items. An example of a training intervention study is that of Danish health care workers by Ibler and colleagues[27] They conducted a randomized clinical trial of education and individual counseling in health care workers with hand eczema. At a 5-month follow-up visit they found a decrease in hand eczema severity score, the primary outcome, and also an improved life-quality index, improved score for self-evaluated severity, and improved skin protective behavior (hand washing and wearing gloves) but no change in knowledge of hand eczema. They also conducted a long-term follow-up at 42 to 47 months and at that time found no significant differences between the control and intervention groups.[28] They suggested that the educational intervention needed to be repeated periodically to be effective. Two recent cluster randomized trials of programs addressing dermatitis in health care workers found modest improvements.[29,30] A Dutch study of a skin care program including the provision of cream dispensers found no significant differences between the intervention and control groups although there were some positive effects.[29] A study in the United Kingdom examined a behavioral change package plus the provision of moisturizing creams. Although the odds ratio for hand dermatitis was 0.7 in the intervention compared with the control group, this was not significant and the investigators concluded that there was insufficient evidence to say that the intervention was effective.[30] The various training programs that have been described in working populations have been summarized by Zack and colleagues.[31]

A series of studies have examined prevention practices in the workplaces of workers being assessed for possible OSD.[32–35] The results of these studies are summarized in **Table 1**, and the findings demonstrate a significant gap in training, particularly for skin protection even though legislation in Ontario, Canada where these studies have been conducted requires general and job-specific and Workplace Hazardous Materials Information System training. Although there has been improvement over time, there are still significant gaps in training.

## SCREENING

If primary prevention strategies are not implemented or fail, the use of screening may be important. Diseases for which screening is appropriate should be common, have an early symptomatic stage, have a simple to use and acceptable screening test, and have treatments that improve outcomes.

OSD is common. Several studies have demonstrated improved outcome with early detection.[36–39] Holness studied outcomes of 76 workers with hand dermatitis at a 6-month follow-up assessment and found that improvement in dermatitis was related to the duration of the dermatitis before their definitive assessment.[36] For those who had their dermatitis for less than 12 month before assessment, 53% had improved, whereas for those with dermatitis greater than 12 months only 23% had improved. Hald and colleagues[37] assessed 333 patients 6 months after diagnosis. They found that the odds ratio of a poor prognosis increased by a factor of 1.1 per month of patient delay and 1.05 per month of health care delay. Malkonen and colleagues[38] studied a group of 605 patients with occupational hand eczema followed-up between 7 and 14 years and found that the duration of hand eczema before diagnosis was the most significantly associated factor with healing. The odds ratio for those with 1 to 2 years of eczema before diagnosis was 2.05, whereas the odds ratio for those with a duration of greater than 10 years was 4.55. Adisesh and colleagues[39] reported on a group of 510 cases reported to EPIDERM. They found that those who did not improve had been exposed to the causative agent for a longer period of time (7.6 years) compared with those who did improve (5.3 years).

Given the evidence that OSD is common and early detection improves outcomes, Nichol and colleagues[22] have developed a simple screening tool that can be administrated by occupational health professionals or used for self-screening. The tool

Table 1
Workplace prevention practices reported by workers being assessed for occupational skin disease in Ontario workplaces over time

| | 2000 (%)[32] | 2010 (%)[33] | 2014 (%)[34] | 2016 (%)[35] |
|---|---|---|---|---|
| General occupational health and safety training | 68 | 77 | 81 | 80 |
| Workplace Hazardous Materials Information System training | 58 | 84 | 80 | 76 |
| Skin-specific training | 34 | — | 49 | 39 |
| Avoid exposure | — | — | 87 | 77 |
| Glove use | 45 | 44 | 78 | 75 |
| Hand washing | 35 | — | 92 | 75 |
| Skin care/creams | — | 31 | 34 | 28 |
| Warning signs | — | 31 | 34 | 32 |

Data from Refs.[32–35]

includes questions about dermatitis and exposure characteristics and a visual guide with descriptions that identify normal, mild, or moderate-to-severe changes. In the validation study of 508 health care workers in Ontario, 225 were screened by an occupational health nurse and 283 self-screened. In total 30.5% screened positive, 28% of those screened by an occupational health nurse and 32.5% of those who self-screened. The evaluation of the screening tool was positive, with 99% finding it easy to use and 94% noting it took less than 2 minutes to perform. Eighty-six percent thought workplace screening was very important.

## DIAGNOSIS
### Diagnostic Criteria

As many occupational diseases, the diagnosis of OCD and OCU consists of diagnosing the disease and then establishing the work relatedness of the disease. Mathias outlined diagnostic criteria for OCD in 1989.[40] The criteria are presented in **Box 1**. Two groups have evaluated the Mathias criteria, one in Israel and one in Spain.[41,42] Ingber and Merins studied a small group of 19 patients.[41] Gomez de Carvallo et assessed 103 patients.[42] The patients were assessed by 2 individuals, one a dermatologist based on their usual clinical practice and the other by an independent specialist using the Mathias criteria. The prevalence of OCD was 11.65%. The dermatologist identified 12 patients and the Mathias criteria identified 13, resulting in a sensitivity of 100% and specificity of 98.9%.[42] The Mathias criteria are commonly used as the basis for diagnosis. A similar set of questions for OCU has been proposed (**Box 2**).[43]

### Clinical Testing

To determine whether the OCD or OCU is allergic in nature, patch testing is used for ACD and a variety of tests of OCU. Patch testing methodology is well described in a

---

**Box 1**
**Mathias criteria for the diagnosis of work-related skin disease**

1. Is the clinical appearance consistent with contact dermatitis?

2. Are there workplace exposures to potential cutaneous irritants or allergens?

3. Is the anatomic distribution of the dermatitis consistent with the form of cutaneous exposure in relation to the job task?

4. Is the temporal relationship between exposure and onset consistent with contact dermatitis?

5. Are nonoccupational exposures excluded as likely causes?

6. Does removal from exposure lead to improvement of the dermatitis?

7. Do patch tests or provocation tests implicate a specific workplace exposure?

Additional criteria that may be used to evaluate *aggravation* of contact dermatitis:
1. Has new dermatitis occurred on skin surfaces not previously affected by preexisting dermatitis?
2. Has dermatitis become more severe on skin surfaces already affected by preexisting dermatitis even though no new skin surfaces are involved?

*From* Mathias CG. Contact dermatitis and workers' compensation: criteria for establishing occupational causation and aggravation. J Am Acad Dermatol 1989;20(5 Pt 1):842-8; with permission.

---

**Box 2**
**Criteria for the diagnosis of occupational contact urticaria**

1. Documentation of the clinical diagnosis of urticaria has been made by medical examination.

2. The workplace agent thought to be the possible cause has been documented in medical or toxicologic studies as a potential cause of urticaria.

3. The timing of the cutaneous allergen exposure and the urticarial response should be in keeping with an immediate hypersensitivity reaction.

4. Symptoms and the site of urticaria should be consistent with the route of exposure to the presumed causal workplace agent.

5. The temporal relationship between the urticaria and the workplace exposure should include complete resolution on weekends, vacations or other times when the worker has left the workplace, and should only occur in the workplace.

6. Other non–work-related causes of urticaria have been excluded.

7. The causal relationship between the workplace exposure and urticaria has been confirmed with medical testing.

*Adapted from* Holness DL, Arrandale VH, Pacheco K, Malo J-L, Bernstein DI. Occupational urticaria and allergic contact dermatitis. In Asthma in the Workplace 4th edition, in press.

---

primer by Lachapelle and Maibach.[44] In addition to screening sets of patch test haptens, there are several commercially available sets of haptens that are specific to particular occupations or agents such as rubber, epoxy, and dental, and these should be used when investigating a possible occupational OACD. In addition to commercially prepared haptens, testing with workplace agents is also possible. The process is described in the work by Lachapelle and Maibach.[44] Care must be taken when doing testing with workplace agents and should only be done by practitioners who have expertise in patch testing and OCD. The value of testing with workplace agents has been demonstrated for several allergens including epoxy and isocyanates.[45,46]

For OCU, there are several possible methods including open controlled application, skin prick testing, or a closed patch test for 20 minutes.[47] Prick testing is described in the primer by Lachapelle and Maibach.[44] Unlike patch testing where there are hundreds of available commercial haptens for testing, there are fewer extracts for skin prick testing. The most commonly available are foods. Serum-specific IgE and RAST tests can also be used for some allergens.

## MANAGEMENT
### Medical Management

The management of both OCD and OCU consists of both medical management and also management of the workplace. The medical management has been well described in several recent guidelines such as Johnston and colleagues for contact dermatitis and Zuberbier and colleagues and Magerl and colleagues for contact urticaria.[2,47,48] These will not be reviewed here in detail, as the clinician should use current clinical guidelines and best practices in medical management.

In the case of work-related disease, workplace management is very important because if you do not eliminate the causative exposure, no matter how good the medical management, the results may be limited if the workplace exposures are not dealt with. The workplace management considerations are outlined in the next section on return to work.

### *Return to Work*

To some extent, workplace management for return to work is applying the primary prevention strategies again. Particular attention is focused on reducing or eliminating the exposure depending on the mechanism. For allergic contact dermatitis or contact urticaria, the worker may have to be removed from exposure to the causative agent, whereas for irritant contact dermatitis a reduction in exposure may be the intervention. In addition, ensuring appropriate personal protective equipment and skin care are important in workplace return and management. The use of glove liners and ensuring the appropriate use of emollients are important factors to consider.[25]

Good communication is needed to ensure both the worker and workplace have clear instructions for workplace modifications. In a follow-up study of 75 workers who were assessed 3 months following diagnosis return to work communication was limited.[49] Only 23% reported that their physician wrote a letter to employer regarding their return to work. To fill this gap, a standardized template "The Workplace Prescription" (**Fig. 1**) was developed.[50] It is a tool that is easy to use and provides written directions for aspects of prevention including avoidance of exposure (total avoidance or limited times of exposure) and instructions on glove use (type and use of glove liners) and appropriate skin care.

There is scant information about return to work programs or their outcomes. The approach to return to work for nurses working in health care is described by Chen and colleagues.[51] In addition to the items already mentioned, for workers with OICD, there may need to be a gradual return to work with increasing hours until

St. Michael's
Inspired Care.
Inspiring Science.

WORKPLACE RECOMMENDATIONS FOLLOWING DERMATOLOGY ASSESSMENT©

Patient's Name: ____________ Physician: ____________ Date: ____________

| EXPOSURE MODIFICATIONS | | SKIN CARE MANAGEMENT SUGGESTIONS | | |
|---|---|---|---|---|
| NO Exposure | O ____<br>O ____<br>O ____<br>O ____ | Hand Washing | **What to Use**<br>O alcohol hand rubs<br>O non-foaming cleanser<br>O lukewarm water<br>O Other (specify): | **Additional Information**<br>O Cetaphil Cleanser<br>O CeraVe Cleanser<br>O rinse /dry thoroughly (including spaces between fingers)<br>O avoid wearing rings<br>O refer to allergen information sheets |
| REDUCE as much as possible | O wet work<br>O prolonged glove use (>20 minutes)<br>O fragranced products<br>O harsh products for hand washing (gritty soaps, solvents, etc.)<br>O mechanical irritation (friction, trauma, heavy use of hands, etc.)<br>O extreme heat or cold<br>O Other (specify): | Treatment | O moisturizer<br>O skin diary<br>O follow up with physician if worsens | O apply before work<br>O apply after each break<br>O apply after work<br>O apply after each hand washing<br>O CeraVe Moisturizing Cream<br>O CeraVe Moisturizing Lotion<br>O Cetaphil ____<br>O Prevex<br>O Other (specify): |
| | | | O prescribed medication | |
| Workplace Modifications | O return-to-work/stay-at-work with no changes<br>O return-to- work /stay-at-work with modifications<br>O return-to-work with graduated # of hours: ____<br>O maximum # of back-to-back shifts: ____ | Gloves | O single-use (disposable)<br>O multi-use (re-useable)<br>O cotton liner<br>O nitrile<br>O natural rubber/latex<br>O vinyl<br>O accelerator-free<br>O anti-impact<br>O other (specify): | O hands should be clean prior to donning gloves<br>O discard after each use<br>O discard at first sign of damage<br>O discard at first sign of sweating<br>O discard after 20 minutes<br>O review donning/doffing techniques<br>O N-Dex Free<br>O Other: |
| | Other strategies:<br>O reduce duration of exposure (eg., job rotation)<br>O use of long-handled tools (eg., brush, sponge, scoops etc.)<br>O Other: | Other Personal Protective Equipment | O protective arm sleeves<br>O disposable gown/coveralls<br>O face shield | |

Department of Occupational & Environmental Health, 4th Floor Shuter Wing, 30 Bond St., TORONTO, Ontario M5B 1W8 (tel): 416 864 5074 (fax): 416 864 5421

**Fig. 1.** The "workplace prescription", St Michael's Hospital Occupational Medicine Clinic.

the threshold for irritant effects occurs. There are useful recommendations for work restrictions related to patient care for health care workers in the Public Health Ontario document.[25]

## OUTCOMES

There are a variety of outcomes to consider including disease, functional, work, quality of life, and insurance.

### Disease Outcomes

Disease outcomes vary, with some workers having complete resolution of their disease and others having ongoing problems despite significant interventions. Nicholson and colleagues[3] reported that similar proportions of workers reported either ongoing symptoms or recovery. Nethercott and Holness reported on the disease outcomes of 201 workers with OCD who were assessed again on average 4 years postdiagnosis and found that 76% reported improvement and 40% were free of symptoms.[52] Nicholson and colleagues[3] note there is little information available related to OCU.

### Functional Outcomes

There is limited information about objective functional outcomes in workers with OCD. Holness and colleagues[53] studied a group of 62 workers and assessed their hand and upper extremity function from several perspectives. Physical examination revealed that 57% had some restriction in movement. This included 30% with moderate to severe restriction of their ability to tuck their fingers and 23% with restriction of opposition of the thumb. Eighty-two percent had impairment of grip strength.

### Work

Work outcomes are a nuanced item. Generally, if studies report work outcomes, they are reported simply as number with lost time or working (yes or no). Nicholson and colleagues[3] note that up to half of workers report losing time from work because of their skin disease. In the study by Holness and colleagues,[53] 35% reported missing some work in the preceding year with a mean of 12 weeks of missed work. As to work status, Nicholson and colleagues[3] note that job loss or a change of employment is common. Holness carried out a detailed assessment of 75 workers at 3 and 6 months postdiagnosis.[49] At 6-month follow-up 38% were not working, almost all because of their skin problem. Of the 62% that were working 67% had changed jobs and again almost all because of their skin disease. In a more recent study, Holness and colleagues[53] found that 19% were working at a different job and 9% were not working because of their skin disease. Work productivity and work instability were also examined. Almost half of the workers had moderate-to-high job instability and 31% indicated a loss of productivity of greater than 10% with an average loss of productivity of 8%. In a longer term follow-up of 230 workers with OCD who were followed-up for at least 2 years and on average 4 years, 78% were working but 57% had changed jobs, 67% of these because of their skin.[54]

### Quality of Life

There is a substantial literature on quality of life in workers with OSD. Different tools to assess quality of life have been used, making it more challenging to compare across studies of workers with OSD and when comparing with other dermatologic conditions. Some studies have used generic instruments such as the SF-36 and/or dermatology-specific instruments. The European Academy of Dermatology and Venereology Task

Forces on Quality of Life and Patient Oriented Outcomes and Occupational Skin Disease recommend using the SF36 as a generic instrument for health-related quality of life and the DLQI for dermatology-specific quality of life.[55] They also note the need to study quality of life in OSDs other than OCD.

Most studies have documented an adverse on quality of life.[3] As an example, Holness and colleagues[53] used both the SF36 and the Dermatology Life Quality Index (DLQI) in their detailed functional assessment of 63 workers with suspected OSD. They found that there was more impact on the SF36 mental score than the physical score. On the DLQI, 47% of the workers scored more than 10, consistent with a very large to extremely large effect on dermatologic quality of life.

There have been studies examining mental health in workers with occupational hand dermatitis. In addition to assessing 122 patients with hand dermatitis with the SF36 and the DLQI, Boehm and colleagues[56] also assessed anxiety and depression. They found that 22% had a positive anxiety score and 14% had a positive depression score.

### Use of Insurance or Workers' Compensation

Another outcome that is of importance to the worker is whether they receive monetary compensation for their work illness or work absence. The insurance systems vary from country to country with some having mandatory state-run workers' compensation systems, some having private, voluntary systems, and some using a general disability insurance scheme. These variations make it difficult to compare across jurisdictions. A key issue is whether workers (or their employer depending on the jurisdiction) submit a workers' compensation claim.

### Costs of Occupational Skin Disease

Diepgen and colleagues[57] examined the cost of occupational hand dermatitis in Germany. In a group of 151 with patients with hand OCD, they found that 63% had been absent from work with an average days lost of 76 in the past 12 months. They calculated the cost of 8799 Euros per worker.

In summary, OCD results in functional and quality-of-life deficits to workers, is very costly, and is currently best addressed by screening and early diagnosis and treatment.

### CLINICS CARE POINTS

- For workers exposed to wet work, even if you think it is OICD, it is important to patch test the worker, as they may also have OACD.

- It is useful to patch test with not only a screening tray but also with a tray specific to the occupation or exposure (eg, hairdressing, epoxy).

- Only those with expertise should patch test with chemicals the come from the workplace.

- Management must include not only medical management but also recommendations about removing or reducing exposure to the causative workplace agent and the appropriate gloves and hand care regimen to be used on return to work.

- For those with OICD, a gradated return to work (ie, gradually increasing the hours of work) may be helpful.

### DISCLOSURE

Dr L. Holness holds research grants funded by public granting agencies.

## REFERENCES

1. Lachapelle J-M. Historical aspects. In: Rycroft RJG, Menne T, Frosch PJ, et al, editors. Textbook of contact dermatitis. Berlin: Springer-Verlag; 1992. p. 7.
2. Zuberbier T, Aberer W, Asero R, et al. The EAACI/GA$^2$LEN/EDF/WAO guideline for the definition, classification, diagnosis and management of urticaria. Allergy 2018;73(7):1393–414.
3. Nicholson PJ, Llewellyn D, English JS, et al. Evidence-based guidelines for the prevention, identification and management of occupational contact dermatitis and urticaria. Contact Dermatitis 2010;63(4):177–86.
4. Burnett CA, Lushniak BD, McCarthy W, et al. Occupational dermatitis causing days away from work in US private industry, 1993. Am J Ind Med 1998;34(6):568–73.
5. Morse T. Occupational disease in Connecticut, 2017 2017.
6. Horwitz IB, Kammeyer J, McCall BP. Workers' compensation claims related to natural rubber latex gloves among Oregon healthcare employees from 1987 to 1998. BMC Public Health 2002;2:21.
7. Malerich PG, Wilson ML, Mowad CM. The effect of a transition to powder-free latex gloves on workers' compensation claims for latex-related illness. Dermatitis 2008;19(6):316–8.
8. Aalto-Korte K, Koskela K, Pesonen M. 12-year data on skin diseases in the Finnish Register of Occupational Diseases I: Distribution of different diagnoses and main causes of allergic contact dermatitis. Contact Dermatitis 2020;82(6):337–42.
9. Pesonen M, Koskela K, Aatlo-Korte K. Contact urticaria and protein contact dermatitis in the Finnish Register of Occupational Diseases in a period of 12 years. Contact Dermatitis 2020;83(1):1–7.
10. McDonald JC, Beck MH, Chen Y, et al. Incidence by occupation and industry of work-related skin diseases in the United Kingdom, 1996-2001. Occup Med (Lond) 2006;56(6):398–405.
11. Pal TM, de Wilde NS, van Beurden MM, et al. Nottiication of occupational skin diseases by dermatologists in The Netherlanss. Occup Med (Lond) 2009;59(1):38–43.
12. Turner S, McNamee R, Agius R, et al. Evaluating interventions aimed at reducing occupational exposure to latex and rubber glove allergens. Occup Environ Med 2012;69(12):925–31.
13. Stocks SJ, McNamee R, Turner S, et al. The impact of national-level interventions to improve hygiene on the incidence of irritant contact dermatitis in healthcare workers: changes in incidence from 1996 to 2012 and interrupted time series analysis. Contact Dermatitis 2015;173(1):165–71.
14. Bensefa-Colas L, Telle-Lamberton M, Faye S, et al. Occupational contact urticaria: lessons learned from the French National Network for Occupational Disease Vigilance and Prevention (RNV3P). Br J Dermatol 2015;173(6):1453–61.
15. Carder M, Bensefa-Colas L, Mattiolo S, et al. A review of occupational disease surveillance systems in Modernet countries. Occup Med (Lond) 2015;65(8):615–25.
16. Rietschel RL, Mathias CGT, Fowler JF, et al. Relationship of occupation to contact dermatitis: evaluation in patients tested from 1998 to 2000. Am J Contact Dermatitis 2002;13(4):170–6.
17. Pesonen M, Jolanki R, Larese Filon F, et al. Patch test results of the European baseline series among patients with occupational contact dermatitis across

Europe - analyses of the European Surveillance System on Contact Allergy network, 2002-2010. Contact Dermatitis 2015;72(3):154–63.

18. Higgins CL, Palmer AM, Cahill JL, et al. Occupational skin disease among Australian healthcare workers: a retrospective analysis from an occupational dermatology clinic, 1993-2014. Contact Dermatitis 2016;75(4):213–22.

19. Ibler KS, Jemec GBE, Flyvholm MA, et al. Hand eczema: prevalence and risk factors of hand eczema in a population of 2274 healthcare workers. Contact Dermatitis 2012;67(4):200–7.

20. Lan CCE, Tu HP, Lee CH, et al. Hand dermatitis among university hospital nursing staff with or without atopic eczema: assessment of risk factors. Contact Dermatitis 2011;64(2):73–9.

21. Luk NMT, Lee HCS, Luk CKD, et al. Hand eczema among Hong Kong nurses: A self-report questionnaire survey conducted in a regional hospital. Contact Dermatitis 2011;65(6):329–35.

22. Nichol K, Copes R, Kersey K, et al. Screening for hand dermatitis in healthcare workers: comparing workplace screening with dermatologist photo screening. Contact Dermatitis 2019;80(6):374–81.

23. Ibler KS, Jemec GBE, Garvey LH, et al. Prevalence of delayed-type and immediate type hypersensitivity in healthcare workers wth hand eczema. Contact Dermatitis 2016;75(4):223–9.

24. Aerts O, Dendooven W, Foubert K, et al. Surgical mask dermatitis caused by formaldehyde (releasers) during the COVID-19 pandemic. Contact Dermatitis 2020;83(2):172–3.

25. Public Health Ontario, Civedino M, Holness DL, Smith J, et al. Recommendations for the prevention, detection and management of occupational contact dermatitis in healthcare workers. Public Health Ontario 2019.

26. Bauer A, Ronsch H, Elsner P, et al. Interventions for preventing occupational irritant contact dermatitis. Cochrane Database Syst Rev 2018;4(4):CD004414.

27. Ibler KS, Jemec GBE, Diepgen TL, et al. Skin care education and individual counselling versus treatement as usual in healthcare workers with hand eczema: randomized clinical trial. BMJ 2012;345:e7822.

28. Graversgaard C, Agner T, Jemec GBE, et al. A long term followup study of the Hand Eczeema Trial (HET): a randomized clinical trial of a secondary preventive programme introduced to Danish healthcare workerrs. Contact Dermatitis 2018; 78(5):329–34.

29. Soltanipoor M, Kezic S, Sluiter JK, et al. Effectiveness of a skin care programme for the prevention f contact dematitis in helathcare workers (the Healthy Hands Project): a single-centre, cluster randomized trial. Contact Dermatiits 2019; 80(6):365–73.

30. Madan I, Parsons V, Ntani G, et al. A behaviour change package to prevent hand dermatitis in nurses working in the National Health Service: results of a cluster randomized controlled trial. Br J Dermatol 2020;183(3):461–70.

31. Zack B, Arrandale VH, Holness DL. Preventing occupational skin disease: a review of training programs. Dermatitis 2017;28(3):169–82.

32. Holness DL, Kudla I. Workers with occupational contact dermatitis: Workplace characteristics and prevention activities. Occup Med (Lond) 2012;62(6):455–7.

33. Rowley K, Ajami D, Gervais D, et al. Glove use and glove education in workers with hand dermatitis. Dermatitis 2016;27(1):30–2.

34. Gupta T, Arrandale VH, Kudla I, et al. Gaps in workplace education practices for prevention of occupational skin disease. Ann Work Expo Health 2018;62(2): 243–7.

35. Zack B, Arrandale V, Holness DL. Skin specific training experience of workers being assessed for contact dermatitis. Occ Med (Lond) 2018;68(3):203–6.
36. Holness DL. Health care services use by workers with work-related contact dermatitis. Dermatitis 2004;15(1):18–24.
37. Hald M, Agner T, Blands J, et al. on behalf of the Danish Dermatitis Group. Delay in medical attention to hand eczema: a follow-up study. Br J Dermatol 2009; 161(6):1294–300.
38. Mälkönen T, Alanko K, Jolanki R, et al. Long-term follow-up study of occupational hand eczema. Br J Dermatol 2010;163(5):999–1006.
39. Adisesh A, Meyer JD, Cherry NM. Prognosis and work absence due to contact dermatitis. Contact Dermatitis 2002;46(5):273–9.
40. Mathias CG. Contact dermatitis and workers' compensation: criteria for establishing occupational causation and aggravation. J Am Acad Dermatol 1989;20(5 Pt 1):842–8.
41. Ingber A, Merins S. The validity of the Mathias criteria for establishing occupational causation and aggravation of contact dermatitis. Contact Dermatitis 2004;51:9–12.
42. Gomez de Carvallo M, Calvo B, Benach J, et al. Assessment of the Mathias Criteria for establishing occupaitonal causation of contact dermatitis. Actas Dermosilfologr 2012;103(5):411–21.
43. Holness DL, Arrandale VH, Pacheco K, et al. Occupational urticaria and allergic contact dermatitis. In Asthma in the workplace 4th edition, in press.
44. Lachapelle JM, Maibach HI. Patch testing and prick testing. 3rd edition. Berling: Springer; 2020.
45. Houle M, Holness DL, DeKoven J, et al. Additive value of patch testing custom epoxy materials from the workplace at the Occupational Disease Specialty Clinic in Toronto. Dermatitis 2012;23(5):214–9.
46. Burrows D, Houle M-C, Holness DL, et al. Additive value of patch testing custom isocyanate materials from the workplace at the Occupational Disease Specialty Clinic in Toronto. Dermatitis 2015;26(2):94–8.
47. Magerl M, Altrichter S, Borzova E, et al. The definition, diagnostic testing, and management of chronic inducible urticarias - The EAACI/GA(2) LEN/EDF/UNEV consensus recommendations 2016 update and revision. Allergy 2016;71(6): 780–802.
48. Johnston GA, Exton LS, Mohd Mustapa MF, et al. British Association of Dermatologists' guidelines for the management of contact dermatitis. Br J Dermatol 2017; 176(2):317–29.
49. Holness DL. Workers with occupational contact dermatitis: work outcomes and return to work process in the first six months following diagnosis. J Aller (Cairo) 2011;2011:170693.
50. Kudla I, Houle M-C, Velykoredko Y, et al. Introducing a "workplace prescription" to facilitate return to work for workers with occupational contact dermatitis. J Cutan Med Surg 2017;21(6):573–5.
51. Chen J, Gomez P, DeKoven J, et al. Return to work for nurses with hand dermatitis. Dermatitis 2016;27(5):308–12.
52. Nethercott JR, Holness DL. Disease outcome in workers with occupational skin disease. J Am Acad Dermatol 1994;30(4):569–74.
53. Holness DL, Harniman E, DeKoven J, et al. Hand and upper extremity function in workers with hand dermatitis. Dermatitis 2013;24(3):131–6.
54. Holness DL, Nethercott JR. Work outcome in workers with occupational skin disease. Am J Ind Med 1995;27(6):807–15.

55. Chernyshov PV, John SM, Tomas-Aragones L, et al. Quality of life measurement in occupational skin disease. Position paper of The European Academy of Dermatology and Venereology Task Forces on quality of life and patient oriented outcomes and occupational skin disease. J Eur Acad Dermatol Venereol 2020. https://doi.org/10.1111/jdv.16742.
56. Boehm D, Schmid-Ott G, Finkeldey FF, et al. Anxiety, depression and impaired health-related quality of life in patients with occupational hand eczema. Contact Dermatitis 2012;67(4):184–92.
57. Diepgen TL, Scheidt R, Weisshaar E, et al. Cost of illness from occupational hand eczema in Germany. Contact Dermatitis 2013;9(2):99–106.

# Identifying Safe Alternatives for Contact Allergy Patients

Andrew Scheman, MD[a],*, Elise Fournier, BS[b], Lilly Kerchinsky, BS[b], Jason Wei, BS[c]

## KEYWORDS

- Contact allergy alternatives • Contact dermatitis alternatives • Allergy alternatives
- Allergen alternatives • Safe alternatives for contact allergy
- Safe alternatives for contact dermatitis • Contact allergy safe products
- Contact dermatitis safe products

## KEY POINTS

- Allergen avoidance is the most effective treatment of contact allergy.
- Patient improvement ultimately relies on identification of safe alternative products, which can be used by the patient.
- This article discusses specific safe alternatives for the 80 allergens on the 2017 American Contact Dermatitis Society core allergen series.

## TOPICAL AND HOUSEHOLD PRODUCTS

Allergen avoidance is the most effective treatment of individuals with allergic contact dermatitis (ACD). Many allergens in topical and household products, however, have multiple names and cross-reactors (CRs), which make them difficult to avoid when reading product labels. In addition, some products may be labeled "unscented" or "fragrance free," yet use fragrance ingredients to mask underlying aromas or contain fragranced essential oils that contain allergenic fragrance chemicals. The American Contact Dermatitis Society (ACDS) created the Contact Allergen Management Program (CAMP) to help individuals find safe alternatives.[1] CAMP can be programmed specifically to avoid each patient's allergens, allergen synonyms, and CRs. Physicians who join the ACDS can use the CAMP app to find safe alternatives for skin, hair, cosmetic, and household products for their patients. Member physicians can go to the ACDS CAMP Web site, click boxes corresponding to each substance to which

[a] Northwestern University Feinberg School of Medicine, 420 E Superior St, Chicago, IL 60611, USA; [b] Michigan State University, 426 Auditorium Rd, East Lansing, MI 48824, USA; [c] University of Illinois Urbana-Champaign, 1304 W Pennsylvania Ave, Urbana, IL 61801, USA
* Corresponding author. 1535 Lake Cook Road, Suite 401, Northbrook, IL 60062.
E-mail address: patchtest@scheman.com

Immunol Allergy Clin N Am 41 (2021) 455–466
https://doi.org/10.1016/j.iac.2021.05.001
0889-8561/21/© 2021 Elsevier Inc. All rights reserved.
immunology.theclinics.com

their patient is allergic, and then click "generate search codes" to obtain individualized codes for their patient. Patients then can download the ACDS CAMP app (Apple or Android) for free, and type in their user codes to have an easily searchable list of safe skin, hair, cosmetic, topical medication, laundry, dish, and household products with them at all times.

## ISSUES WITH SPECIFIC ALLERGENS IN TOPICAL AND HOUSEHOLD PRODUCTS

There are some unique issues to consider when finding safe alternatives for certain contact allergens. These issues are discussed.

### Corticosteroids

Finding alternatives for patients with steroid allergy is challenging because of their anti-inflammatory properties, which may mask positive reactions on a patch test. If a patient is found allergic to 1 type of steroid, there still may be others that are masked by a false-negative reaction.

Steroids have been divided into structural groups A, B, C, D1, and D2.[2] Contact allergy occurs most commonly with groups A, B, and D2 steroids[3] and these are combined into 1 CR group in CAMP. The other 2 steroid CR groups in CAMP are structural group C and structural group D1. If an individual is allergic to a steroid in 1 CR group, CAMP suggests alternative steroids from the other CR groups. If the patient also is allergic to preservatives or other vehicle ingredients, CAMP suggests steroids that also are free of these ingredients. Unfortunately, many exceptions exist with steroid CRs. Therefore, when CAMP suggests a potentially safe alternative steroid, this should be double-checked by having the patient perform a repeat open application test by applying the proposed steroid to the volar forearm twice daily for 2 weeks with a Q-Tip or similar cotton swab to ensure no reaction occurs before using elsewhere on the body.[4]

Alternatively, a patient's physician can try prescribing a nonsteroidal anti-inflammatory topical medication, such as tacrolimus, pimecrolimus or crisaborole.

If systemic or injectable steroids are required, the most likely safe alternatives are oral dexamethasone (dexamethasone, 1.5 mg = prednisone, 10 mg) and injectable betamethasone.

### Hair Dye

Para-phenylenediamine (PPD) is the most common allergen found in hair dyes. It is used in dyes to help achieve darker natural colors. Patients who are allergic to PPD may cross-react with methylated PPD and para-toluenediamine sulfate.[5,6] Testing the patient to a full hair dye tray indicates which hair dye ingredients are safe alternatives. Schwarzkopf Igora Royal or Goldwell Top Chic are alternatives for patients allergic only to PPD. Light Mountain Natural Hair Dye is safe to use if allergic only to PPD and its derivatives.

### Chlorhexidine

Povidone-iodine or ethanol-based scrubs are possible alternatives for patients with allergy to chlorhexidine. Safe topical products free of this allergen can be found on the CAMP app, similar to other product types.

## METHYLISOTHIAZOLINONE/METHYLCHLOROISOTHIAZOLINONE

Found in many topical and household products, the allergens methylisothiazolinone/methylchloroisothiazolinone are also are in most US interior acrylic wall paints and glues.[7,8] Methylisothiazolinone/methylchloroisothiazolinone in interior acrylic paints may remain airborne in high-enough concentrations to cause allergic reactions for up to 5 weeks or more.[9]

### Nail Products

Nail polishes often contain tosylamide/formaldehyde resin (also known as toluene sulfonamide formaldehyde resin). Products with alternative resins can be found using CAMP. Nail glues typically contain ethyl cyanoacrylate. Individuals allergic to this allergen must avoid nail glues. No-chip, acrylic, gel, and dip nail products must be avoided by those allergic to acrylates and/or methacrylates; safe nail polishes without acrylates can be found using CAMP.

### Oral Allergens

Some allergens are known to cause oral mucosal contact allergies. Balsam of Peru constituents are used in some artificial flavoring and also are found naturally in some foods. Patients allergic to balsam of Peru can be placed on a balsam-restricted diet.[10]

Avoidance diets have been published for other oral allergens and causes of systemic contact allergy, such as nickel, cobalt, chromate, propylene glycol, benzoic acid, sorbic acid, and formaldehydes.[11–14] Systemic allergy occurs when ingestion of an allergen reactivates dermatitis at the site of previous contact allergy by stimulation of memory T cells at the site which recognizes this particular allergen.

Lauryl (dodecyl) gallate is used as an antioxidant in margarine and many cooking oils. Butter and extra-virgin olive oil are safe alternatives.[14] Benzoyl peroxide is used to bleach flour. Unbleached flour is a safe alternative. Both of these allergens typically are destroyed when heated, making them safe for allergic individuals to consume.[15,16] Therefore, the main relevant exposure to lauryl gallate is salad and sandwich dressings. The main relevant food exposure to benzoyl peroxide is rolls and pizza dipped in raw bleached flour after cooking; however, heating these foods in an oven before eating likely renders them safe.

### Compositae

Patients with contact allergy to Compositae (Asteraceae) plants should be aware that they may not only cause reactions by direct contact, but also from airborne exposure. Several patch test allergens indicate Compositae allergy, including Compositae mix, sesquiterpene mix, and parthenolide. There are more than 32,000 species of Compositae plants. Airborne allergy is challenging because there is no easy way to totally avoid airborne exposure to these allergens. Some Compositae also are ingested and are known to cause systemic contact allergy (ie, chamomile tea, lettuce, sunflower seeds, and bay leaves).[17] Safe topical products free of this allergen can be found on the CAMP app, similar to other product types.

### Formaldehyde

Formaldehyde-allergic patients should avoid topical products with formaldehyde-releasing preservatives (quaternium-15, DMDM hydantoin, imidazolidinyl urea, diazolidinyl urea, and 2-bromo-2-nitropropane-1,3-diol).[18] Also, most keratin treatments contain formaldehyde (often using an alternative chemical name). Formaldehyde often is found (in varying concentrations) in clothlike paper goods (cotton/paper blends) even if not listed as an ingredient (eg in wipes, fabric softener sheets, and clothlike paper towels).[19,20] For this reason, fabric softener sheets likely should be avoided by formaldehyde-allergic patients even if listed as "safe" in CAMP. Wipes and clothlike paper towels should be avoided or gloves worn when handling these items.

### Benzalkonium Chloride

Benzalkonium chloride is used as an antimicrobial agent as well as a preservative. It is found in most antimicrobial wipes, sprays, and solutions. It is safest to wear gloves when handling these products. A safe alternative is to use bleach (60 mL) or chlorine pool chemical (30 mL) per liter of water with paper towels. Safe topical products free of this allergen can be found on the CAMP app, similar to other product types.

### Colophony

Colophony (rosin) is a sticky substance derived from pine trees.[21] Safe alternatives are found using CAMP. Colophony also is found in many household products, such as adhesives and various home repair products (varnish, polishes, paints, caulk, and so forth). It is safest to use gloves when handling these products. Colophony also is an ingredient used to make recycled paper. It is safest to choose plastic bags for groceries.

## OTHER COMMON ALLERGENS

CAMP is not helpful for finding alternative for allergens not found in topical or household products. Finding alternatives for other common allergens is discussed later.

### Nickel

ACD to nickel is common. Patients can detect and avoid nickel in everyday products. A nickel test kit is recommended to identify objects (such as door handles, jewelry, and keys) that should be avoided. A list of sources to obtain nickel test kits can be found in **Table 1**.[22]

For keys, brass is a safe alternative. Allergenic handles can be coated with Krylon Clear Acrylic Spray.[23] For jewelry, platinum, sterling silver, and yellow gold are safe alternatives. White gold can be coated with platinum or rhodium by a jeweler. Aside from brass and bronze, most metal costume jewelry should be avoided.

The American Contact Alternatives Group (ACAG) has published a list of specific nickel-free alternative products.[22]

Patients should be made aware that nickel can be transferred to sensitive areas (such as the face) through passive transfer from the hands.

### Cobalt

Identifying cobalt can be done using a cobalt test kit (Chemotechnique, Vellinge, Sweden).[24] Cobalt is found in some steel alloys, notably objects plated with nickel. It also is found in some white gold. Some common objects that cobalt may be found in include jewelry, children's toys, antiqued jewelry (typically a zinc-cobalt alloy), blue paints, and art materials. Perhaps the most common source of cobalt exposure is its increasing use to tan fine leather.[24,25]

### Potassium Dichromate

If individuals are found allergic to potassium dichromate, they need to avoid hexavalent chromium, which often is used to tan fine leather. These patients should avoid direct contact with tanned leather. Hexavalent chromate also is found in some Portland cement. Allergic patients also should avoid eye cosmetics with chromium green pigments. The ACDS CAMP app can identify safe alternative products.

| Table 1 | | | |
|---|---|---|---|
| Nickel spot test kits | | | |
| Web Site | Size | Price | Link |
| Etsy | 10 mL | $10.24 | https://www.etsy.com/listing/541231831/nickel-spot-test-testing-kit-tester?ga order=most relevant&ga search type=all&ga view type=gallery&ga search query=nickel %20spot%20kit&ref=sr gallery-1-1&organix search click=1 (or, search nickel spot kit on Etsy) |
| Delasco | 0.5 oz | $19.00 | https://www.delasco.com/pcat/1/Chemicals/Spot Test for Nickel Kit/dlmin009?/ |
| NoNickel.com | 0.23 oz | $24.95 | https://nonikel.com/products/nickel-alert-nickel-test-kit |
| Smart Practice | 10 swabs | $19.99 | http://www.smartpractice.com/Apps/WebObjects/ SmartPractice.woa/wa/style?id=DMAL8003&m=|SPA |

*From* Scheman A, Jacob SE, Nedorost S, Katta R et al. Alternatives for allergens in the 2018 American Contact Dermatitis Society core series: report by the American Contact Alternatives Group. Dermatitis 2019:30:87-105; with permission.

## Gold

Exposure to gold can be from dental fillings or jewelry. Individuals with oral mucosal reactions to a gold (or other metal) filling can replace it with fillings made from acrylates/methacrylates. Due to passive transfer from the hands, reactions to gold also may occur on sites of the body not directly in contact with gold (especially the face).[26] To prevent this reaction, gold jewelry can be coated with rhodium or platinum.

## Shoes

Individuals allergic to various materials found in shoes should wear shoes free of these allergens until their condition clears then can reintroduce 1 pair of shoes per week to determine which are tolerated. New shoes also should be introduced 1 per week to identify any which cause a problem. If a patient is having reactions limited to the soles, sometimes simply replacing the insole with a safe material will be sufficient. If a patient is allergic to rubber accelerators, colophony or paratertiary butylphenol formaldehyde resin, a shoe repair store first should remove any adhesive used to glue the insole in place. A list of shoes free of various allergens is found in **Table 2**.[22]

## Textile Dyes

Disperse dyes most often are the cause of clothing ACD. These types of dyes are used primarily on synthetic fabrics, so direct skin contact with nonwhite clothing made from polyester, acrylic, acetate, or nylon (including cotton/synthetic blends) should be avoided.

## Textile Finishes

Most modern clothing no longer uses textile finish resins, which release reactive amounts of free formaldehyde.[27]

Vintage clothing and older clothing containing cotton and/or rayon should be avoided. Cotton and/or rayon upholstery still may contain older formaldehyde textile resins and these chemicals also are used in fiberboard and home insulation.

## Oeko-Tex Labeling

Certain European fabrics are certified by Oeko-Tex to be free of disperse dyes and formaldehyde textile resins. These fabrics are acceptable for individuals with allergies to textile resins and dyes.

**Table 2**
Shoe allergens

| Shoe Type | Brand | Leather | Chromates | Cobalt | Paratertiary Butylphenol Formaldehyde Resin | Colophony | Thiurams | Carbamates | Benzothiazoles | Thioureas | Lack Rubber |
|---|---|---|---|---|---|---|---|---|---|---|---|
| Boot | Wesco Boots | Yes | No | No | No | No | No | No | No | No | No |
| | Multnomah Leather Shop | Yes | No | No | No | No | No | No | No | No | No |
| | Loveless Shoes | Yes | No | No | No | No | No | No | No | No | No |
| Sandal | Crocs (plastic copolymer) | No | No | No | No | No | No | No | No | No | No |
| | Birkenstock (cork foot, EVA sole, Birkibuc) | No | No | No | No | No | No | No | No | No | No |
| | Juju Footwear (plastic) | No | No | No | No | No | No | No | No | No | No |
| | Jellies (plastic) | No | No | No | No | No | No | No | No | No | No |
| Casual | Beyond Skin (vegan and wide varieties) | No | No | No | ? | ? | No | No | No | No | No |
| | TOMS (canvas upper) | No | No | No | No | Yes | PO | PO | PO | PO | PO |
| | SeaVees (canvas upper, cotton insole) | No | No | No | ? | ? | ? | ? | ? | ? | ? |
| Gym | Allbirds (wool, recycled plastic bottles, and recycled cardboard) | No | No | No | No | ? | No | No | No | No | No |
| | Saucony[a] | No (unless leather upper) | No (unless leather upper) | No (unless leather upper) | No | No | PO | PO | PO | PO | PO |
| Work | Servus Injection Molded Footwear (PVC with steel toe protection) | No | No | No | No | No | No | No | No | No | No |

Abbreviation: ?, information on this allergen was omitted by the manufacturer; EVA, Ethylene Vinyl Acetate; PO, probably OK; PU, Polyurethane; PVC, Polyvinyl Chloride.

[a] Saucony—look at the description of the shoe to determine if safe to use. It is recommended to choose a shoe with an EVA or PU midsole.

From Scheman A, Jacob SE, Nedorost S, Katta R et al. Alternatives for allergens in the 2018 American Contact Dermatitis Society core series: report by the American Contact Alternatives Group. Dermatitis 2019;30:87-105; with permission.

## Leather

Potassium dichromate and cobalt chloride are the most common allergens relevant to the tanning of fine leather. Also, paratertiary butylphenol formaldehyde resin is used as a leather adhesive. Allergic individuals may react to leather found in clothing, shoes, belts, bags, or furniture. The best treatment of these patients is leather avoidance or vegan leather.

## Adhesives

General household adhesives often contain a variety of materials that may cause ACD, including colophony, acrylates/methacrylates, cyanoacrylates, rubber-related allergens, epoxies, and isocyanates (polyurethane adhesives). There usually is more than 1 acceptable type of adhesive for most tasks, and the safest approach is to choose an alternative glue based on a material to which the patient is not allergic. **Table 3** shows appropriate adhesive choices for various tasks.[22]

### Bandage Adhesives

Acrylic and rubber-related adhesives are the most likely causes of ACD due to bandages. The best alternatives are bandages with silicone adhesives because allergy and irritation to silicone adhesives is extremely uncommon.[22] For home bandages, a suitable alternative is Curad Truly Ouchless Flexible Fabric Bandage. For medical tape, suitable alternatives include 3M Spunlace Polyester Nonwoven Fabric Medical Tape or Vancive medical single-coated duolaminate polyurethane film tape with soft silicone adhesive (product number: MED 5500SI). Additionally, for a bandage dressing, a suitable alternative is Pderm High Adhesion Silicone Gel Adhesive Coated Polyurethane Film.

### Eyelash Adhesives

False eyelashes and eyelash extensions contain rubber, cyanoacrylate, or methacrylate/acrylate adhesive. In false eyelashes, Duo Eyelash Adhesives (black or white) contain rubber-based adhesive, Novalash contains cyanoacrylate, and those that contain methacrylate/acrylate adhesives include House of Lashes, Velour Lashes, and Duo Brush-On Striplash Adhesive. Lash Professional eyelash extensions contain cyanoacrylate. Individuals with reactivity to 1 or more of these allergens should use 1 of the other products listed or may use growth products, such as bimatoprost ophthalmic solution (Latisse).[22]

### Electrocardiogram Electrode Adhesives

Electrocardiogram electrode pad adhesives may contain acrylates (3M Electrically Conductive Cushioning Gasket Tape, and Vermed SofTouch ECG Electrode), silicone (3M XYZ-axis Electrically Conductive Transfer Tape), or rubber-related compounds (3M High Permeability Magnetic Shielding Sheet 1380). If an individual has a known ACD to 1 of these materials, 1 of the other electrodes listed may be used.[22]

### Dental Adhesives

Individuals with allergies to acrylates/methacrylates must inform their dentist or orthodontist of their condition because many materials used in dentistry contain these materials. Patients with acrylate/methacrylate allergy can react to these materials; however, the risk can be reduced by using cotton rolls (to prevent gum contact) and rinsing out residual unhardened monomer. Also, curing time should be extended. Once fully hardened (ie, polymerized), these materials are less likely to cause allergy.

**Table 3**
**General household adhesives**

| Bonding Surface | Glue Types | Products |
|---|---|---|
| Ceramics | Acrylate | Elmer's Craft Bond Ceramic and Glass Cement |
| | Epoxy | Elmer's Fiberglass Repair System |
| | Cyanoacrylate | Krazy Glue–quick setting |
| | Synthetic rubber | Elmer's Professional Contact Cement |
| | | Elmer's Heavy Duty Grip Cement |
| | Polyurethane | Gorilla Glue |
| Fabric | Polyvinyl acetate based | Elmer's Glue-All—all-purpose white glue |
| | Rubber based | Elmer's Craft Bond Rubber Cement |
| | Polyurethane | Gorilla Glue |
| Glass | Cyanoacrylate | Krazy Glue–quick setting |
| | Polyurethane | Gorilla Glue |
| | Acrylate | Elmer's Craft Bond Ceramic and Glass Cement |
| | Epoxy | Elmer's Fiberglass Repair System |
| Metal | Cyanoacrylate | Krazy Glue–quick setting |
| | Epoxy | Loctite Quick-Set Epoxy |
| | Synthetic rubber | Elmer's Professional Contact Cement |
| | | Elmer's Heavy Duty Grip Cement |
| Organic | Acrylate | Elmer's Craft Bond Ceramic and Glass Cement |
| | Cyanoacrylate | Krazy Glue–quick setting |
| | Polyurethane | Gorilla Glue |
| | Rubber based | Elmer's Craft Bond acid-free spray |
| | Epoxy | Loctite Quick-Set Epoxy |
| Paper | Polyvinyl acetate based | Elmer's Glue-All—all-purpose white glue |
| | Acrylate | Elmer's Craft Bond Ceramic and Glass Cement |
| | Polyurethane | Gorilla Glue |
| | Rubber Based | Elmer's Craft Bond acid-free spray |
| | Cyanoacrylate | Krazy Glue–quick setting |
| Plastic | Polyvinyl acetate based | Elmer's Glue-All—all-purpose white glue |
| | Synthetic rubber | Elmer's Professional Contact Cement |
| | Cyanoacrylate | Krazy Glue–quick setting |
| | Epoxy | Loctite Quick-Set Epoxy |
| | Rubber based | Elmer's Craft Bond acid-free spray |
| | Polyvinyl acetate based | Elmer's Glue-All—all-purpose white glue |
| Wood | Synthetic rubber | Elmer's Professional Contact Cement |
| | | Elmer's Heavy Duty Grip Cement |
| | Polyvinyl acetate based | Elmer's Glue-All—all-purpose white glue |
| | Epoxy | Elmer's Wood Repair |
| | | Elmer's Superfast Epoxy Cement |

From Scheman A, Jacob SE, Nedorost S, Katta R et al. Alternatives for allergens in the 2018 American Contact Dermatitis Society core series: report by the American Contact Alternatives Group. Dermatitis 2019:30:87-105; with permission.

### Rubber Accelerators

Patients who patch test positive for carbamates, thirurams, benzothiazoles, or thioureas have ACD to rubber accelerators. Rubber accelerators are used in the manufacturing of rubber materials, such as examination gloves, rubber bands, and other common objects, to speed up the process of vulcanization. Unfortunately, companies that make rubber and artificial rubber objects are not required by law to list the

**Table 4**
**Accelerator-free gloves (free of thiurams, carbamates, benzothiazoles, thioureas, diphenylguanidine, and latex protein)**

| Medical Examination Gloves | | | |
| --- | --- | --- | --- |
| Company | Ordering | Web Site | Products |
| Ansell Healthcare | 1-855-868-5540 | www.ansell.com | Microflex Sensation Nitrile Exam, Micro-Touch NitraFree Nitrile Exam |
| Cardinal Health | 1-800-964-5227 | www.cardinalhealth.com | Low Dermatitis Potential Nitrile Exam |
| Dynarex Corporation | 1-888-396-2739 | www.dynarex.com | Tillotson True Advantage Nitrile Exam Gloves |
| Hourglass International | 1-800-277-0994 | www.hourglass-intl.com | HandPRO FreeStyle1100 Nitrile Exam |
| Sempermed USA | 1-800-366-9545 | www.sempermedusa.com | SemperSure Nitrile Exam |
| SmartPractice | 1-800-365-6868 | www.smartpractice.com | Reflection Sapphire Sensitive Nitrile PF Violet Blue |

| Surgical Gloves | | | |
| --- | --- | --- | --- |
| Company | Ordering | Web Site | Products |
| Ansell Healthcare | 1-855-868-5540 | www.ansell.com | GAMMEX® Non-Latex Polyisoprene Surgical Glove, GAMMEX Non-Latex Sensitive Synthetic Sensoprene Surgical Glove |
| Medline Industries, Inc. | 1-800-633-5463 | www.medline.com | DermAssure Green Powder-Free Neoprene Surgical Glove |
| Mölnlycke Health Care US LLC | 1-800-843-8497 | www.molnlycke.com | Biogel NeoDerm Neoprene Surgical Glove |

| Household and Industrial Gloves | | | | | |
| --- | --- | --- | --- | --- | --- |
| Company | Ordering | Web Site | Product | Purpose | Type |
| Allerderm | 1-800-365-6868 | www.myskinallergy.com | Allerderm Heavy Duty Vinyl Gloves | Cleaning, dishes | Reusable |
| Showa Group | 1-800-241-0323 | www.showagroup.com | N-Dex 9500 PF Nitrile | Longer, thicker nitrile glove | Disposable |
| Showa Group | 1-800-241-0323 | www.showagroup.com | 7712 PVC | Chemical protection; (chemical list on Showa Web site) | Reusable |
| Honeywell | 1-800-234-7437 | www.fishersci.ca | Honeywell North Silver Shield/4H Gloves | Extremely chemical resistant | Reusable |

*From* Scheman A, Jacob SE, Nedorost S, Katta R et al. Alternatives for allergens in the 2018 American Contact Dermatitis Society core series: report by the American Contact Alternatives Group. Dermatitis 2019;30:87-105; with permission.

specific rubber accelerators used to make the products. Some objects may have multiple accelerators present.

For medical and household gloves, accelerator-free alternatives are listed in **Table 4.**[22]

Patients also may react to rubber household objects. For patients allergic to rubber makeup applicators, it is possible to use Q-Tips, cotton balls, or brushes to apply products. Clothing items that may contain rubber include swimwear, undergarments, and socks. For swimwear, safe alternatives are made by Decent Exposures and Rawganique. Decent Exposures and Cottonique make accelerator-free undergarments (bras and both men and women's underwear). For socks, Cottonique makes latex-free adult booties and Elite Elastic-free 100% Cotton Socks. For condoms, LifeStyles Healthcare North America makes Skyn Original Condoms, which are polyurethane-free and latex-free and protect against human immunodeficiency virus transmission.

### Rubber in Sports Protective Equipment

Rubber accelerators can be found in certain sports and exercise equipment. Certain objects, such as earplugs, athletic tape, mouth guards, and support braces, may need to be considered for the presence of rubber accelerators. BioSkin supports and braces are safe for patients to use. Specific swim, soccer, and basketball equipment alternatives have been published by the ACAG.[22]

For sports that require protective equipment, such as hockey or football, a prosthetic or orthotic maker can apply a protective polyurethane foam that creates a barrier between the allergenic product and a patient's skin.

### CLINICS CARE POINTS

- After patch testing identifies allergens to avoid, safe alternative products must be identified.
- Physicians should have knowledge of safe alternatives to treat contact allergy patients successfully.
- Contact allergy treatment success improves with hands-on patient education regarding allergen avoidance and safe alternatives.

### DISCLOSURE

The authors have nothing to disclose.

### REFERENCES

1. Scheman A, Severson D. American contact dermatitis society contact allergy management program: an epidemiologic tool to quantify ingredient usage. Dermatitis 2016;27:11–3.
2. Jacob SE, Steele T. Corticosteroid classes: a quick reference guide including patch test substances and cross-reactivity. J Am Acad Dermatol 2006;54:723–7.
3. Baeck M, Chemelle J-A, Rasse C, et al. C(16)-methyl corticosteroids are far less allergenic than the non-methylated molecules. Contact Derm 2011;64:305–12.
4. Chang Y-C, Clarke GF, Maibach HI. The provocative use test (PUT) [repeated open application test (ROAT)] in topical corticosteroid allergic contact dermatitis. Contact Derm 1997;37:309–11.

5. Scheman A, Cha C, Bhinder M. Alternative Hair-Dye Products for Persons Allergic to para-Phenylenediamine. Dermatitis 2011;22:189–92.

6. Schuttelaar M, Dittmar D, Burgerhof JGM, et al. Cross-elicitation responses to 2-methoxymethy-p-phenylenediamine in p-phenylenediamine-allergic individuals: Results from open use testing and diagnostic patch testing. Contact Derm 2018;79:288–94.

7. Goodier MC, Siegel PD, Zang L-Y, et al. Isothiazolinone in Residential Interior Wall Paint: A High-Performance Liquid Chromatographic-Mass Spectrometry Analysis. Dermatitis 2018;29:332–8.

8. Goodier MC, Zang L-Y, Siegel PD, et al. Isothiazolinone Content of US Consumer Adhesives: Ultrahigh-Performance Liquid Chromatographic Mass Spectrometry Analysis. Dermatitis 2019;30:129–34.

9. Christiansen MS, Agner T, Ebbehøj NE. Long-lasting allergic contact dermatitis caused by methylisothiazolinone in wall paint: A case report. Contact Derm 2018;79:112–3.

10. Salam TN, Fowler J Jr. Balsam-related systemic contact dermatitis. J Am Acad Dermatol 2001;45:377–81.

11. Mislankar M, Zirwas J. Low-Nickel Diet Scoring System for Systemic Nickel Allergy. Dermatitis 2013;24:190–5.

12. Stuckert J, Nedorost S. Low-cobalt diet for dyshidrotic eczema patients. Contact Derm 2008;59:361–5.

13. Sharma AD. Low Chromate Diet in Dermatology. Indian J Dermatol 2009;54:293–5.

14. Scheman A, Cha C, Jacob SE, et al. Food Avoidance Diets for Systemic, Lip, and Oral Contact Allergy: An American Contact Alternatives Group Article. Dermatitis 2012;23:248–57.

15. Youssef S. Evaluation of antioxidants stability by thermal analysis and its protective effect in heated edible vegetable oil. Ciênc Tecnol Aliment 2011;31:475–80.

16. Lazar M, Ambrovic P. Thermal Decomposition of Benzoyl Peroxide in Solid State. Chem Zvesti 1969;23:881–94.

17. Paulsen E. Systemic allergic dermatitis caused by sesquiterpene lactones. Contact Dermatitis 2016;76:1–10.

18. De Groot A, White IR, Flyhom M. Formaldehyde-releasers in cosmetics: relationship to formaldehyde contact allergy. Part 2. Patch test relationship to formaldehyde contact allergy, experimental provocation tests, amount of formaldehyde released, and assessment of risk to consumers allergic to formaldehyde. Contact Derm 2010;62:18–31.

19. Liou YL, Ericson ME, Warshaw EM. Formaldehyde Release From Baby Wipes: Analysis Using the Chromotropic Acid Method. Dermatitis 2019;30:207–12.

20. Piletta-Zanin P-A, Pache-Koo F, Auderset PC, et al. Detection of formaldehyde in moistened baby toilet tissues. Contact Derm 1998;38:46.

21. Jackson JD, Helms SE. Gums, rosin, and natural resins. 7th edition. Fischer's Contact Dermatitis; 2019. p. 541–56.

22. Scheman A, Hylwa-Deufel S, Jacob SE, et al. Alternatives for Allergens in the 2018 American Contact Dermatitis Society Core Series: Report by the American Contact Alternatives Group. Dermatitis 2019;30:87–105.

23. Herro EM, Jacob SE, Scheman A. Nickel Exposure From Household Items: Potential Method of Protection. Dermatitis 2012;23:188–90.

24. Thyssen JP, Menné T, Johansen JD, et al. A spot test for detection of cobalt release - early experience and findings. Contact Derm 2010;63:63–9.

25. Bregnbak D, Thyssen JP, Zachariae C, et al. Association between cobalt allergy and dermatitis caused by leather articles – questionnaire study. Contact Derm 2014;72:106–14.
26. Fowler J Jr, Taylor J, Storrs F, et al. Gold Allergy in North America. Am J Contact Dermatitis 2001;12:3–5.
27. De Groot AC, Maibach HI. Does allergic contact dermatitis from formaldehyde in clothes treated with durable-press chemical finishes exist in the USA? Contact Derm 2010;62:127–36.

# Contact Urticaria

Ana M. Gimenez-Arnau, MD[a],*, Howard Maibach, MD[b]

## KEYWORDS

- Contact urticaria • Dermatitis • Eczema • Immediate contact reaction • Immunology
- Protein contact dermatitis • Syndrome • Urticaria

## KEY POINTS

- Immediate contact skin reactions constitute the chronic urticaria syndrome and usually appear within minutes after contact with eliciting substances.
- In the occupational setting chronic urticaria syndrome seems to be common, although it is difficult to obtain in most countries because of underreporting.
- The same substance can induce different clinical patterns, opening the door for new insights into immune system pathways.

Until now it was assumed that new cases of contact urticaria (CoU) were exceptional findings; each year added new substances to long lists of triggers. But is this condition really exceptional? CoU is an important clinical manifestation and part of the contact urticaria syndrome (CUS). CoU still is often underdiagnosed or misdiagnosed. Clinicians should disseminate knowledge of this entity among their medical colleagues, among patients, and among health authorities involved in occupational health. CoU impairs daily activities and quality of life, and can be life-threatening, but if it is correctly diagnosed it can be prevented and successfully treated.

The concept of contact dermatitis includes any inflammatory skin reaction to direct or indirect contact with noxious agents in the environment. Although the main clinical expression of contact dermatitis is eczema, CoU and lichenoid eruptions are also described. The earliest recorded reports include Pliny the Younger who, in the first century AD, noticed individuals with severe itching when cutting pine trees. Patch and prick testing are considered the main tools for discovering the responsible agent.

In the last decades, it has been learned that proteins and low-molecular-weight (LMW) molecules can induce immediate cutaneous reactions (ICSR).

## CONTACT URTICARIA AND CONTACT URTICARIA SYNDROME

CUS comprises a heterogeneous group of ICSR reactions that usually appear within minutes after contact with eliciting substances. Occasionally systemic involvement

[a] Department of Dermatology, Hospital del Mar, Universitat Autònoma de Barcelona, Passeig Maritim 25-29, Barcelona 08021, Spain; [b] Department of Dermatology, University of California, San Francisco, 90 Medical Center Way, San Francisco, CA 9413, USA
* Corresponding author.
E-mail address: anamariagimenezarnau@gmail.com

Immunol Allergy Clin N Am 41 (2021) 467–480
https://doi.org/10.1016/j.iac.2021.04.007
0889-8561/21/© 2021 Elsevier Inc. All rights reserved.
immunology.theclinics.com

is present. Maibach and Johnson[1] defined it as an entity in 1975. Since then its scientific interest has increased, and new cases are continuously reported, providing information concerning new trigger factors and clinical features.

CoU refers to a wheal and flare reaction following external contact with a substance, usually appearing within 30 minutes and clearing completely within hours, without residual signs.[2] Fisher[3] introduced the term in 1973, but this phenomenon has long been recognized. Urticarial lesions to nettles and hairy caterpillars were reported in the nineteenth century and continue being reported today.[4] In a survey carried out in 1224 adults in Spain, contact wheals and pruritus were noticed by 52.1% and 100%, respectively, of people who suffered cutaneous symptoms induced by the pine processionary moth.[5] Naturally occurring urticariogens were used therapeutically as rubefacients, counterirritants, and also vesicants.[6]

In 1976, Hjorth and Roed-Petersen defined protein contact dermatitis (PCD) as an immediate dermatitis induced after contact with proteins.[7-9] Thirty-three food caterers suffering exacerbation of itch immediately after contact with meat, fish, and vegetables followed by erythema and vesicles were described. Application of the relevant foods to the affected skin resulted in either urticaria or eczema.[10] Atopy and PCD are associated in approximately 50% of affected patients.[11]

Patients suffering CUS can develop CoU and/or dermatitis/eczema immediately after the contact with the trigger substance. These ICSR can appear on normal or eczematous skin, can be induced by the same trigger factor, and can be suffered by the same patient.

## EPIDEMIOLOGY AND OCCUPATIONAL RELEVANCE OF CONTACT URTICARIA

It is unlikely that CoU is rare, especially among individuals with atopy, but no figures on its prevalence in the general population are available. The global incidence of CUS is not known. ICSR are common in dermatologic practice.[9,12-16] With the exception of natural rubber latex (NRL) allergy, trigger factors for only isolated cases or short series of patients are described.[11] The symptoms of CoU are usually mild, of short duration, and limited to small skin areas. The diagnostic tests are rarely performed, because neither patients nor physicians are interested in the mechanisms of these minor symptoms. Thus, the probable diagnosis of CoU is seldom recorded in patient files. General knowledge on the epidemiology of CoU is largely based on the statistics of certain countries that register occupational cases of CoU.

NRL caused an epidemic of occupational CoU in health care workers in the 1990s because of escalating glove use in this sector.[17] In an international meta-analysis from studies performed in 1990 to 2003, IgE-mediated allergy to NRL ranged from 1.4% to 1.65% in the general population, and from 4.1% to 5% in the health care worker population.[18] New cases of NRL allergy have decreased significantly, especially after health authorities have required the use of low-allergen/low-protein nonpowdered protective gloves. The prevalence of immediate NRL allergy in Western Europe is approximately 1% or less.[18]

There are limited data on the prevalence of ICSR other than NRL allergy. Skin contact reactions are a part of the clinical spectrum of many common immediate-type hypersensitivity reactions, providing that the skin is exposed to a significant extent to the allergen in question. This is probably not the case with airborne allergens, such as pollen, but other allergens, such as animal dander and excretions, cause skin contact reactions.

Some hints of the prevalence of CoU are found in the literature, although skin symptoms are seldom reported in larger series of immediate allergy. About one-third of birch pollen sensitive patients also react to cross-reactive fruit and vegetables. In 1977, Hannuksela and Lahti[19] reported skin contact symptoms in a series of 152 patients allergic to birch pollen who also reacted to at least two different allergens in a scratch-chamber test of 25 different fruits and vegetables. Of the 52 patients who reacted to raw potato, 17 had itching and/or urticaria-like edema of the hands after peeling potatoes; of the 59 apple-positive patients 4 had itchy dermatitis of the hands after handling apples, and of the 46 carrot-positive patients 6 had similar symptoms after peeling carrots.[19] In a Spanish series of 197 children with IgE-mediated fish allergy, 29 children had cutaneous symptoms after skin contact with fish.[20] Peach allergy is another example of an immunologic hypersensitivity reaction whose clinical spectrum includes skin reactions. Among 30 patients allergic to peach in Northern Spain, there were six cases of CoU.[21] Authors of the study did not comment on whether or not the CoU cases were occupational. In Australia, peanut butter under an occlusive dressing was applied to the healthy skin of 281 children who were prick-test-positive to peanut. A total of 114 of the children had an urticaria reaction.[22]

In the occupational setting CUS seems to be common, although a precise statistical analysis is difficult to obtain in most of the countries because of underreporting. In a few countries, CoU has been classified as a separate occupational skin disease. This is the case in Finland since 1989. The Finnish Register of Occupational Diseases (1990–1994) showed that CoU was the second most frequent cause of occupational dermatosis (29.5%), after contact allergic dermatitis (70.5%).[23,24] The trigger agents were cow dander (44.4%); NRL (23.7%); and flour, grains, or feed (11.3%).[25] A smaller proportion of occupational CoU was found in a retrospective study done in a tertiary-level clinic specializing in occupational dermatology in Melbourne, Australia, showing an 8.3% CoU prevalence.[26] Hands, arms, and face were the most frequent body area involved. Atopy was a significant risk factor for NRL, foodstuffs, or ammonium persulfate CoU. Health workers, food handlers, and hairdressers were the most common occupations affected. More recently, a survey conducted in 335 restaurant, catering, and fast-food employees in Singapore showed occupational irritant contact dermatitis was more common (10%) with CoU reported in only two patients, caused by lobster and prawn.[27] The nature of the exposure probably determines the percentage of CoU risk.

Consultant dermatologists in the United Kingdom report occupational skin diseases to EPIDERM, a voluntary surveillance system. Occupational physicians have a similar scheme called OPRA. In 1996 to 2001, most cases of CoU were attributed to rubber materials or foods and flour. CoU was diagnosed particularly in the health and social services and in food and organic material manufacturing.[28] In EPIDERM, CoU was relevant in 4% of the cases of occupational skin disease. In accordance with the Australian data, the rates for CoU among women were twice those among men. In 2002 to 2005, the number of CoU cases reported to EPIDERM was 336; 41% of these were codiagnosed with contact dermatitis, and 75.5% were associated with exposure to NRL.[29] When data from EPIDERM and OPRA were combined, cases of CoU peaked in 1996, but have since declined.[30] According to the Finnish Register of Occupational Diseases, in 2005 to 2010 there were 329 (10.4%) notified as occupational cases of CoU or PCD among a total of 3170 notified cases of occupational skin disease. These figures are comparable with the Australian data. The earlier Finnish statistics only comprised suspected cases, and the number of notified cases was not available. The number of CoU and/or PCD cases seems to have decreased. In 1990 to 1994 the number of suspected new cases was 815 (an average of 163 suspected cases/year),[24] whereas in 2005 to 2010 there was only an average of 74 new suspected cases/year. In line with the Australian and the UK data, as regards the notified cases, CoU and/or PCD was more common among women (62%) than among men (38%). In 2005 to 2010, the most common causes of the notified cases were cow dander (48%), flour, grain or animal feed (17%), NRL (10%), and other food (9%). Because only the primary diagnosis is recorded in the Finnish register, some cases are not registered. This is particularly the case when allergic contact dermatitis is considered more important. Industrial enzymes have lost some of their relative significance when compared with 1990 to 1994 data (1.7% vs 0.7%), but decorative plants have not (1990–1994 [1.6%] vs 2005–2010 [2.2%]). The main risk of industrial enzymes is sensitization of the respiratory tract, and only a small minority of sensitized patients have skin contact reactions.

Most CoU cases are caused by protein-containing organic material, and the mechanism is usually IgE-mediated. Occupational CoU caused by LMW chemicals is rare. In Finland they comprised only about 3% of the notified occupational CoU and PCD cases in 2005 to 2010. The mechanism of chemical-induced CoU is sometimes IgE-mediated, but in most cases the mechanism remains unknown. Ammonium persulfate was the most common LMW chemical, followed by organic acid anhydrides.

Occupational CoU in European health care workers shows a prevalence from 5% to 10%, whereas in the general population it lies between 1% and 3%. Other occupations with a high risk to develop CoU include food handlers or people involved in agriculture, farming, floriculture, plastics, pharmaceutical and other laboratories, hunters, veterinarians, biologists, or hairdressers. Atopy favors further sensitization where protein allergens are concerned.[31]

The classification of occupational dermatosis of the International Classification of Diseases-11 includes contact dermatitis with CoU. Occupational screening questionnaires including specific questions searching for urticaria symptoms are few. The long version of the Nordic Occupational Skin Questionnaire (NOSQ-2002) is one of them including nine questions about urticaria symptoms.[32] A standardized method to evaluate the occupational relevance of CoU, such as the Mathias criteria,[33] already developed for occupational contact dermatitis would be desirable.

Regarding prognosis of occupational CoU, in a 6-month follow-up study of 1048 patients diagnosed with an occupational skin disease at the Finnish Institute of Occupational Health (FIOH), patients with CoU or PCD had the most favorable prognosis compared with those with occupational allergic contact dermatitis and occupational irritant contact dermatitis.[34] This material also comprised patients with CoU as a sole diagnosis. In a recent Danish report on work-related hand dermatoses in food-related occupations, patients with PCD had experienced more severe and frequent consequences than patients with other diagnoses.[35] In Finland, the long-term outcome of NRL allergy was studied in 160 adult patients a median of 3 years after diagnosis. In their working environment, all gloves had been changed to either low-allergen NRL or non-NRL gloves. Not one of 71 health care workers had changed jobs because of NRL allergy, and the prevalence of hand eczema had decreased significantly (54% vs 38%).[36]

## EVOLVING KNOWLEDGE ABOUT THE MECHANISMS INVOLVED IN CONTACT URTICARIA

The mechanisms underlying ICSR are partially understood. Each trigger substance has its own mechanism of action.

Nonimmunologic CoU (NICoU) is caused by vasogenic mediators without involvement of immunologic processes. Urticariogens may act following different patterns. The most classic example concerns dimethyl sulfoxide, which damages the blood vessels, making them leaky and inducing mast cell degranulation.[37] Antihistamines do not inhibit reactions to dimethyl sulfoxide and other NICoU responsible agents, but acetylsalicylic acid and nonsteroidal anti-inflammatory drugs do (orally and topically); therefore, a role for prostaglandins has been suggested.[38–40] Release of prostaglandin $D_2$ without concomitant histamine release has been demonstrated following topical application of sorbic acid and benzoic acid.[41,42] Capsaicin pretreatment (which depletes substance P) does not impair NICoU, but does inhibit the allergen prick test flare of immunologic CoU (ICoU).[43] Nonspecific tachyphylaxis of variable duration has been associated with various urticariogens.[44] Sharp hairs from animals or spines from plants penetrating the skin can deliver a cocktail of irritant chemicals or proinflammatory mediators causing NICoU.[45]

The pathogenesis of ICoU including the oral allergy syndrome reflects a type I hypersensitivity reaction, mediated by allergen-specific IgE in a previously sensitized individual.[46–49] Skin challenge involves allergen penetration through the epidermis; IgE binding on mast cells; its degranulation; and subsequent release of histamine and other vasoactive substances, such as prostaglandins, leukotrienes, and kinins.

A combination of type I and type IV allergic skin reactions, the latter supported by positive delayed patch tests, has been suggested as PCD pathogenesis.[50,51] It has been speculated that PCD is an eczematous IgE-mediated reaction through proteins. PCD shows a similar reaction pattern to aeroallergen-induced atopic eczema or dermatitis.[52]

## CLINICAL MANIFESTATIONS OF CONTACT URTICARIA AND CONTACT URTICARIA SYNDROME

CUS clinical symptoms are determined by the route, duration, and extent of exposure; the inherent sensitizing properties of the allergen; and an individual's genetic and/or acquired susceptibility.

CoU is defined by its primary lesion, which is named wheal or hive. There is transient edema of the dermal tissue and a surrounding reflex erythema with itch or sometimes burning sensation at the same time.[37,53–55] The wheal has a fleeting nature and the skin return to its normal appearance usually within 1 to 24 hours.[53]

CoU belongs to the group of inducible urticarias.[54] CoU is characterized by a local immediate and/or delayed urticarial reaction at sites of epidermal or transdermal contact with certain agents. CoU is the oldest form of urticaria recorded. The association of nettles and urticaria was discussed in the Greek literature more than 2000 years ago.[55]

The clinical appearance of the primary lesion of CoU does not differ from that of other types of urticaria. Depending on the type of contacting the wheal can show different aspects. Nettles of plants habitually cause linearly arranged wheals. Punctate wheals arise exactly at the site where the stinging hairs penetrate the skin. The shape of the wheals can change with time. Intense reactions induce confluent lesions. Wheals can start in a follicular pattern if the contactant penetrates through the hair follicles. The associated local symptoms are tingling, itching, and sometimes burning at the sites of the wheal.

The wheals start with redness at the site of contact, followed by whealing at the same site within 10 to 30 minutes after contact. The maximal size is reached 45 minutes afterward, and within 2 hours, the swelling disappears. Redness can persist even 6 hours, exceptionally more than 24 hours. CoU can reappear after 4 to 5 hours. This dual response has been demonstrated experimentally in the ears of BALB/mice and in humans.[56] Delayed onset of CoU was also described, after repeated applications of the trigger substance.[57] The time course and intensity of CoU lesions differ depending of the nature of the eliciting agent. This variability may also be caused by differences in the reactivity of the cells that secrete the vasoactive amines or the sensitivity of the target tissue to the mediators or chemical released.

Contact-induced angioedema shows a sudden, erythematous or skin-colored swelling of the lower dermis and subcutis with frequent involvement below mucous membranes up to 72 hours.

CUS has been classified in four stages. Stages 1 and 2 show cutaneous symptoms. Stage 1 includes flare reactions, wheals, and eczema, and such symptoms as itching, tingling, or burning sensation. When CoU is present it shows itchy wheals that are usually strictly limited to contact areas and that disappear within a few hours without residual lesions. Chronic paronychia with redness and swelling of the proximal nail fold after handling food[58] and NRL[59] can also be observed in PCD. Stage 2 refers to the development of generalized urticaria after a local contact. Stages 3 and 4 include extracutaneous reactions or symptoms that may also occur as part of a more severe reaction. Stage 3 may include bronchial asthma, rhinoconjunctivitis, orolaryngeal symptoms, or gastrointestinal dysfunctions.[60,61] By contact or in the case of a volatile allergen, rhinoconjunctivitis and asthma may accompany the skin manifestations, as occurs with bakers who are in continuous contact with flour. Abdominal pain, diarrhea, and oral allergy syndrome may develop when the allergen comes in contact with the oropharyngeal mucosa.[37,62] Finally, in stage 4, anaphylactic or anaphylactoid reactions may occur as the most severe type of CUS manifestation. CoU can be life threatening: certain substances, such as latex protein, can induce anaphylaxis and even death.

## DIAGNOSTIC TOOLS USEFUL TO MAKE AN ETIOLOGIC DIAGNOSIS IN CONTACT URTICARIA

Diagnosis of CUS is based on full medical history and skin testing with suspected substances. In vitro techniques are available for only a few allergens, including latex. The simplest cutaneous provocation test for ICoU, NICoU, and immediate contact dermatitis, such as PCD, is the "open test." The suspected substance is applied and gently rubbed on slightly affected skin or on a normal-looking 3 × 3 cm area of the skin, either on the upper back or the extensor side of the upper arm. Often it is desirable to apply contact urticants to skin sites suggested by the patient's history. A positive result is edema and/or erythema typical of CoU. Immunologic and nonimmunologic contact reactions usually appear within 15 to 20 minutes. Nonimmunologic contact reactions tend to resolve within 45 to 60 minutes. ICoU can also show a delayed onset, although this is rare.

When the open test results are negative, "prick testing" of suspected allergens is often the method of choice for immediate contact reactions. "Scratch test" and "chamber scratch test" (contact with a small aluminum chamber for 15 minutes) are less standardized than the prick test, but are useful when a nonstandard allergen must be studied. Histamine hydrochloride serves as the positive control and aqueous sodium hydroxide as negative reference (**Fig. 1**). When other than cutaneous organs are involved, it is important to begin ICoU testing with much diluted allergen concentrations and to use serial dilutions to minimize allergen exposure. When testing with poorly or nonstandardized substances, control tests should be assessed on at least 20 people to avoid false-positive interpretation. Nonsteroidal anti-inflammatory drugs and antihistamines should be avoided because of the risk of false-negative results. Following the recommended protocol is important for minimizing the occurrence of hazardous extracutaneous reactions. Life-threatening reactions have been documented during skin tests; therefore, caution is advised, especially when testing certain occupational substances. Skin tests should be performed only if resuscitation equipment and trained personnel are readily available.[63–65]

Skin tests and specific IgE determinations in the diagnosis of CoU and respiratory disease caused by LMW chemicals are even less standardized. Some chemicals induce IgE-mediated allergy. Open application tests (skin provocations) are planned individually. Commercial prick test substances are not available for chemicals, neither are diagnostic guidelines. Examples of testing procedures are found in the literature,

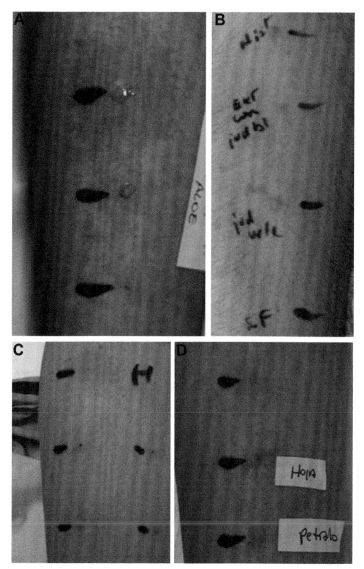

**Fig. 1.** Positive prick tests in patients suffering CoU. In all the cases the upper positive control test is with histamine and the test included below is the negative control with sodium chloride. Induced by (A) positive aloe vera plant, (B) positive green and white bean, (C) positive nitril gloves (twice), and (D) Lilly Stargazer positive leaf stem and petal.

but they usually describe only single cases or small series of cases. Some prick tests were performed with protein conjugates of various LMW chemicals for more than 20 years by the FIOH. Some chemicals can be prick-tested in water solutions, but human serum albumin–hapten conjugates are preferred at FIOH. Prick tests with human serum albumin conjugates are valuable in the diagnosis of immediate acid anhydride allergy (a group of reactive chemicals used in epoxy resin).

Diagnosis of occupational respiratory disease is based on inhalation challenge tests at FIOH.[66]

## AGENTS RESPONSIBLE FOR CONTACT URTICARIA AND THE CONTACT URTICARIA SYNDROME

Proteins (molecular weight 10,000 to several hundred thousands) and also chemicals (molecular weights <1000) can trigger CoU included as an entity in the CUS. Plant or animal proteins, chemicals (eg, drugs and preservatives), or more diverse substances (eg, metals and industrial chemicals) can induce ICoU. LMW molecules normally act as haptens; nevertheless, for some of them IgE antibodies have also been demonstrated, such as sensitized workers reactive to platinum and nickel–serum albumin complexes.[67,68]

NICoU was defined by stinging nettle wheals induced from Urtica dioica. Other responsible agents are preservatives, fragrances and flavorings in cosmetics, toiletries, topical medications, or foodstuffs (eg, benzoic and sorbic acid).[69] Household, industrial, insecticide, and laboratory chemicals can also induce NICoU.

A few substances elicit mixed features of NICoU and ICoU through an unestablished mechanism. In ammonium persulfate–induced CoU, antigen-specific IgG and IgM activate the complement cascade through the classical pathway.[70–72] Immediate reactions to formaldehyde seem not to be mediated by IgE, with a prostaglandin role suspected because of increased levels of thromboxane $B_2$ and prostaglandin $PGF_2$.[73,74]

A huge number of compounds are responsible for occupational and nonoccupational CUS including animal products, plants and plant derivatives, foods, fragrances, cosmetics, flavorings, medications, preservatives, disinfectants, enzymes, metals, and miscellaneous different substances.

NRL allergy focused global interest at the end of the twentieth century. Latex sensitization risk factors include atopy and prolonged exposure via damaged epidermis, such as glove wearers with hand eczema. The 13 allergens of latex better identified and characterized are labeled Hev b1-13. Latex contains approximately 250 polypeptides, 56 of which have been identified as allergens, with a molecular weight of these proteins that varies from 4 to 200 kDa. The antigenic profiles differ between finished products and still raw material. The machining process (eg, the addition of ammonia) can lead to a selective enrichment of chemical and heat-resistant proteins that may be denatured or complexed in new antigenic specificity.[66]

Enzymes are complex proteins or glycoproteins produced by living organisms for the purpose of accelerating biochemical reactions and metabolic processes. Commonly enzymes behave as allergens and are mostly responsible for ICSR mediated by specific IgE antibodies causing CoU and PCD, and the respiratory tract is often involved. Its occupational relevance should always be assessed, and primary preventive measures developed.[66]

Plants in the environment, such as weeds, woods, or ornamentals, cause CUS. ICoU is predominantly found in cultivated plants, whereas toxic or NICoU is most commonly seen in wild plants. Several species of plants have been reported to cause urticaria by unknown/unclassified mechanisms.

Agriculture has high rates of occupational skin diseases reported. Delayed contact allergy commonly occurs from pesticides; however, a scarcity of reports describe pesticide-induced CoU. The present knowledge of CoU to agricultural chemicals, and pesticides in particular, remains deficient.

Direct or indirect skin contact with animals and animal-derived products occurs in numerous occupations, everyday life, and hobbies. Proteins in animal epithelia, excretions, and organs can cause ICoU and NICoU. Individually tailored skin tests for immediate allergy and specific IgE in blood are needed for diagnosing immediate allergy to animals or animal products. Commercial test materials can give false-negative results, thus the skin tests should be made, if possible, with the same materials and in the same format as they have been causing the skin problems.[63]

Food responsible for CUS includes fruits, vegetables, spice, plants, animal proteins, grains, and enzymes. Food additives responsible for CUS include flavoring, fragrances and taste enhancers, preservatives agents, and colorings agents and dyes.[63] Diagnostic tests need to be defined and standardized.

Seminal fluid hypersensitivity is increasingly being recognized as a cause of anaphylaxis and/or intermittent episodic vulvovaginitis. Localized seminal plasma hypersensitivity presents with immediate postcoital vulvovaginal burning, pain, and swelling, rarely associated with vesicles, and can occasionally be present with systemic involvement. It is believed that this condition is more common than recognized. Seminal plasma hypersensitivity is demonstrated with a positive prick test reaction, RAST, and specific RAST inhibition in addition to neutralization of passive transfer antibodies. The most effective treatment approach for women with ICoU seminal plasma hypersensitivity has been immunotherapy.[63]

Topical drugs or, occasionally, systemic drugs that come in contact with the skin or mucosa, may induce CoU, which is often overlooked. Complementary tests (skin tests with immediate readings and, eventually, in vitro tests) are mandatory in certain situations, because a precise diagnosis of the culprit drug and a suggestion of alternative safe drugs is lifesaving. Any drug can induce an ICSR, but most cases have been described with β-lactam antibiotics, topical anesthetics, and, more recently with antiseptics (eg, chlorhexidine).[63]

Cosmetic components can cause CoU with or without systemic symptoms, sometimes life threatening. CUS induced by components included in cosmetics is grossly underdiagnosed and underreported because patients lack awareness. Hair-dye chemicals and bleaches, hair glue, antimicrobial agents and preservatives, fragrance components, toothpaste flavors, botanically derived cosmetic ingredients, permanent makeup and tattoos, and even alcohol are involved as responsible of CUS.[63]

Preservatives and disinfectants are well-documented causes of allergic contact dermatitis, whereas CUS caused by preservatives and disinfectants is less common. It is widely accepted that sodium benzoate, benzoic acid, benzyl alcohol, and sorbic acid cause NICoU and formaldehyde, parabens, povidone-iodine, chloramine, and chlorhexidine can cause ICoU. Preservatives and disinfectants may also cause generalized urticarial, bronchial asthma, rhinitis, conjunctivitis, otolaryngeal and gastrointestinal symptoms, and even anaphylaxis. The mechanism of preservatives (eg, isothiazolinones or formaldehyde releasers) responsible for ICSR is unknown.[63]

Reactive dyes, usually an azo, anthraquinone, or phthalocyanine derivative, show different reactive functional groups to which carrier proteins bind to induce immune responses. Reactive dyes are responsible for CUS stages 1 to 4. Patch testing, prick testing, bronchial challenge tests, and detection of specific IgE to Reactive Dye (RD)-human serum albumin conjugates in serum are used to assess responsible agents, but still need standardization.[66] To establish the relevance between the responsible reactive dyes and their presence in specific textiles is difficult.

Prevalence of CoU from hairdressing products is not fully documented, and only case reports and case series have been published. Hair shampoos, hair conditioners, hair dyes and bleaches, permanent wave preparations, fragrance, and other styling products (eg, sprays, gels, waxes, mousses, lotions, and pomades) have been described as responsible for CUS symptoms. Hairdressers require special education and specific preventive measures.[66]

Despite the frequent exposure to metals, few cases of CoU caused by metals have been reported. The metals involved in CoU are all members of the group called transitional metals (eg, nickel, cobalt, or chromium). Metals are mainly allergenic as salts and not as the metallic form. The mechanism behind CoU caused by metals is unclear, but an IgE-mediated mechanism in indicated because most cases are supported by a positive skin prick test to the metal.[66]

Epoxy resin is commonly used in occupational and nonoccupational setting. The epoxy-resin system includes epoxy resins and other components as curing agents, reactive diluents, modifiers, and additives. Contact dermatitis caused by epoxy resin is often described in the literature, although CoU from epoxy compounds has infrequently been reported and often represents occupational cases. Skin prick test with the patient's "own" epoxy resins aids the diagnosis. Further studies to standardize the diagnostic method are required.[63,66]

## PREVENTION AND TREATMENT OF CONTACT URTICARIA AND CONTACT URTICARIA SYNDROME

Discovering the responsible agent is required to identify the correct avoidance of the eliciting trigger. Avoidance of further exposure improves occupational CoU. Primary and secondary prevention are highly recommended.[75,76] Considering their good safety profile, second-generation antihistamines must be considered the preferred first-line symptomatic treatment of most of CoU.[77] Before considering alternative treatment, higher doses of antihistamines should be used. When dermatitis is present topical immunomodulation is conducted using topical steroids. Severe cases of CUS require a short course of oral steroids or even treatment in an emergency unit.

## CONCLUSIONS AND UNMET NEEDS IN CONTACT URTICARIA

CoU as part of the CUS is a worldwide health problem that needs a global approach. General population-based epidemiologic studies are lacking and are desirable. Structural characteristics of certain proteins and chemicals can induce CoU clinical manifestations through different pathogenic mechanisms. The same substance can induce different clinical patterns. This fact opens the door for new insights into immune system pathways. Substances responsible for ICSR are classified by molecular weight, mechanism of action, occupational relevance, or their common use in daily life. In vivo tests still based on subjective assessment ideally should be replaced by effective in vitro testing for diagnostic purposes. After symptom control, an appropriate etiologic diagnosis and the development of concrete preventive measures is required.

## CLINICS CARE POINTS

- CUS clinical symptoms are determined by the route, duration, and extent of exposure; the inherent sensitizing properties of the allergen; and an individual's genetic and/or acquired susceptibility.

- "Prick testing" of suspected allergens is often the method of choice for immediate contact reactions.

- Discovering the responsible agent is required to identify the correct avoidance of the eliciting trigger; listening to the patient is crucial.

## RECOMMENDED TEXT BOOKS

1. Contact Urticaria Syndrome. Edited by Editors: Giménez-Arnau AM and Maibach H. CRC Press. Boca Raton. New York. 2015
2. Contact Urticaria Syndrome. Diagnosis and Management Editors: Giménez-Arnau AM and Maibach H. Springer 2018

## REFERENCES

1. Maibach HI, Johnson HL. Contact urticaria syndrome: contact urticaria to diethyltoluamide (immediate type hypersensitivity). Arch Dermatol 1975;111:726–30.
2. Wakelin SH. Contact urticaria. Clin Exp Dermatol 2001;26:132–6.
3. Fisher AA. Contact dermatitis. 2nd edition. Philadelphia: Lea & Febiger; 1973. p. 283–6.
4. Lesser E. Lehrbuch der Haut-und Teschlechtskrankheiten Fur studirende und arzte (in German). Leipzig: Verlag von FCW Vogel; 1894.
5. Vega JM, Moneo I, Garcia Ortiz JC, et al. Prevalence of cutaneous reactions to pine processionary moth (Thaumetopoea pityocamba) in an adult population. Contact Dermatitis 2011;64:220–8.
6. Burdick AE, Mathias T. The contact urticaria syndrome. Dermatol Clin 1985;3: 71–84.
7. Maibach HI. Immediate hypersensitivity in hand dermatitis: role of food contact dermatitis. Arch Dermatol 1976;112:1289–91.
8. Hannuksela M. Atopic contact dermatitis. Contact Dermatitis 1980;6:30.
9. Veien NK, Hattel T, Justesen O, et al. Dietary restrictions in the treatment of adult patients with eczema. Contact Dermatitis 1987;17:223–8.
10. Hjorth N, Roed-Petersen J. Occupational protein contact dermatitis in food handlers. Contact Dermatitis 1976;2:28–42.
11. Doutre M-S. Occupational contact urticaria and protein contact dermatitis. Eur J Dermatol 2005;15(6):419–24.
12. Elpern DJ. The syndrome of immediate reactivities (contact urticaria syndrome). An historical study from a dermatology practice. I. Age, sex, race and putative substances. Hawaii Med J 1985;44:426–39.
13. Rudzki E, Rebanel P. Occupational contact urticaria from penicillin. Contact Dermatitis 1985;13:192.
14. Nilsson E. Contact sensitivity and urticaria in "wet" work. Contact Dermatitis 1985; 13:321–8.
15. Turjanmaa K. Incidence of immediate allergy to latex gloves in hospital personnel. Contact Dermatitis 1987;17:270–5.
16. Weissenbach T, Wutrich B, Weihe WH. Allergies to laboratory animals. An epidemiological, allergological study in persons exposed to laboratory animals. Schweiz Med Wochenschr 1988;118:930–8.
17. Palosuo T, Antoniadou I, Gottrup F, et al. Latex medical gloves: time for a reappraisal. Int Arch Allergy Immunol 2011;156:234–46.
18. Bousquet J, Flahault A, Vandenplas O, et al. Natural rubber latex allergy among health care workers: a systematic review of the evidence. J Allergy Clin Immunol 2006;118:447–54.
19. Hannuksela M, Lahti A. Immediate reactions to fruits and vegetables. Contact Dermatitis 1977;3:79–84.
20. Dominguez C, Ojeda I, Crespo JF, et al. Allergic reactions following skin contact with fish. Allergy Asthma Proc 1996;17:83–7.

21. Gamboa PM, Caceres O, Antepara I, et al. Two different profiles of peach allergy in the north of Spain. Allergy 2007;62:408–14.
22. Wainstein BK, Kashef S, Ziegler M, et al. Frequency and significance of immediate contact reactions to peanut in peanut-sensitive children. Clin Exp Allergy 2007;37:839–45.
23. Kanerva L, Jolanki R, Toikkanen J. Frequencies of occupational allergic diseases and gender differences in Finland. Int Arch Occup Environ Health 1994;66:111–6.
24. Kanerva L, Toikkanen J, Jolanki R, et al. Statistical data on occupational contact urticaria. Contact Dermatitis 1996;35:229–33.
25. Kanerva L, Jolanki R, Toikkanen J, et al. Statistics on occupational contact urticaria. In: Amin S, Lahti A, Maibach HI, editors. Contact urticaria syndrome. Boca Raton: CRC Press; 1997. p. 57–69.
26. Williams JD, Lee AY, Matheson MC, et al. Occupational contact urticaria: Australian data. Br J Dermatol 2008;159:125–31.
27. Teo S, Teik-Jin Goon A, Siang LH, et al. Occupational dermatoses in restaurant, catering and fast-food outlets in Singapore. Occup Med (Lond) 2009;59:466–71.
28. Mcdonald JC, Beck MH, Chen Y, et al. Incidence by occupation and industry of work-related skin diseases in the United Kingdom, 1996-2001. Occup Med 2006; 56:398–405.
29. Turner S, Carder M, Van Tongeren M, et al. The incidence of occupational skin disease as reported to The Health and Occupation Reporting (THOR) network between 2002 and 2005. Br J Dermatol 2007;157:713–22.
30. Cherry N, Meyer JD, Adisesh A, et al. Surveillance of occupational skin disease: EPIDERM and OPRA. Br J Dermatol 2000;142:1128–34.
31. Bourrain JL. Occupational contact urticaria. Clin Rev Allergy Immunol 2006;30: 39–46.
32. Susitaival P, Flyvholm MA, Meding B, et al. Nordic occupational skin questionnaire (NOSQ-2002): a new tool for surveying occupational skin diseases and exposure. Contact Dermatitis 2003;49:70–6.
33. Mathias CG. Contact dermatitis and workers' compensation: criteria for establishing occupational causation and aggravation. J Am Acad Dermatol 1989;20: 842–8.
34. Mälkonen T, Jolanki R, Alanko K, et al. A 6-month follow-up study of 1048 patients diagnosed with an occupational skin disease. Contact Dermatitis 2009;61:261–8.
35. Vester L, Thyssen JP, Menne T, et al. Consequences of occupational food-related hand dermatoses with a focus on protein contact dermatitis. Contact Dermatitis 2012;67:328–33.
36. Turjanmaa K, Kanto M, Kautiainen H, et al. Long-term outcome of 160 adult patients with natural rubber latex allergy. J Allergy Clin Immunol 2002;110:S70–4.
37. Von Krogh C, Maibach HI. The contact urticaria syndrome. An update review. J Am Acad Dermatol 1981;5:328–42.
38. Kligman AM. Dimethyl sulphoxide I and II. J Am Med Assoc 1965;193:796–804, 923-928.
39. Lahti A, Oikarinen A, Viinikka L, et al. Prostaglandins in contact urticaria induced by benzoic acid. Acta Dermatol Venereol (Stockh) 1983;63:425–7.
40. Lahti A, Vaananen A, Kokkonen E-L, et al. Acetylsalicylic acid inhibits non-immunologic contact urticaria. Contact Dermatitis 1987;16:133–5.
41. Johansson J, Lahti A. Topical non-steroidal anti-inflammatory drugs inhibit non-immunological immediate contact reactions. Contact Dermatitis 1988;19:161–5.

42. Morrow JD, Minton TA, Awad JA, et al. Release of markedly increased quantities of prostaglandin D2 from the skin in vivo in humans following the application of sorbic acid. Arch Dermatol 1994;130:1408–12.

43. Downard CD, Roberts LJ, Morrow JD. Topical benzoic acid induces the increased synthesis of prostaglandin D2 in humans skin in vivo. Clin Pharmacol Ther 1995;74:441–5.

44. Lundblad L, Lundberg JM, Anggard A, et al. Capsaicin sensitive nerves and the cutaneous allergy reaction in man. Possible involvement of sensory neuropeptides in the flare reaction. Allergy 1987;42:20–5.

45. Lahti A, Maibach HI. Long refractory period after application of one nonimmunologic contact urticaria agents to the guinea pig ear. J Am Acad Dermatol 1985;13:585–9.

46. Lovell CR. Urticaria due to plants. In: Lovell CR, editor. Plants and the skin. 1st edition. Oxford: Blackwell Science Ltd; 1993. p. 29–41.

47. Amaro C, Goossens A. Immunological occupational contact urticaria and contact dermatitis from proteins: a review. Contact Dermatitis 2008;58:67–75.

48. Lahti A, Björksten F, Hannuksela M. Allergy to birch pollen and apple, and cross-reactivity of the allergens studied with. RAST Allergy 1980;35:297.

49. Löwenstein H, Eriksson NE. Hypersensitivity to foods among birch pollen-allergic patients. Allergy 1983;38:577.

50. Dreborg S, Foucard T. Allergy to apple, carrot and potato in children with birch pollen allergy. Allergy 1983;38:167.

51. Kanerva L, Estlander T. Immediate and delayed skin allergy from cow dander. Am J Contact Dermat 1997;8:167–9.

52. Conde-Salazar L, Gonzalez MA, Guimaraens D. Type I and type IV sensitization to Anisakis simplex in 2 patients with hand eczema. Contact Dermatitis 2002;46:361.

53. Czarnetzki B. In: Czarnetzki MB, editor. Basic mechanisms en. New York, Tokyo: Urticaria Springer-Verlag; 1986. p. 5–25. Chapter 2.

54. Zuberbier T, Aberer W, Asero R, et al. The EAACI/GA2LEN/EDF/WAO Guideline for the definition classification, diagnosis and management of Urticaria. The 2013 revision and update. Allergy 2014. https://doi.org/10.1111/all.12313.

55. Czarnetzki B. In: Czarnetzki MB, editor. Basic mechanisms en. Berlin Heidelberg, New York, Tokyo: Urticaria Springer-Verlag; 1986. p. 89–95. Chapter 6.

56. Ray MC, Tharp MD, Sullivan TJ, et al. Contact hypersensitivity reactions to dinitrofluorobenzene mediated by monoclonal IgE anti–DNP antibodies. J Immunol 1983;131:1096–102.

57. Andersen KE, Maiback HI. Multiple application delayed onset urticaria. Possible relation to certain unusual formalin and textile reactions. Contact Dermatitis 1984;10:227–34.

58. Tosti A, Guerra L, Morelli R, et al. Role of foods in the pathogenesis of chronic paronychia. J Am Acad Dermatol 1992;27:706–10.

59. Kanerva L. Occupational protein contact dermatitis and paronychia from natural rubber latex. J Eur Acad Dermatol Venereol 2000;14:504–6.

60. Crisi G, Belsito D. Contact urticaria from latex in a patient with immediate hypersensitivity to banana, avocado and peach. Contact Dermatitis 1993;28:247–8.

61. Jeannet-Peter N, Piletta-Zanin PA, Hauser C. Facial dermatitis, contact urticaria, rhinoconjuntivitis, and asthma induced by potato. Am J Contact Dermat 1999;10:40–2.

62. Morren M, Janssens V, Dooms-Goossens A, et al. alpha-Amylase, a flour additive: an important cause of protein contact dermatitis in bakers. J Am Acad Dermatol 1993;29:723–8.

63. Gimenez-Arnau A, Maurer M, de la Cuadra J, et al. Immediate contact skin reactions, an update of contact urticaria, contact urticaria syndrome and protein contact dermatitis: a never ending story. Eur J Dermatol 2010;20:1–11.

64. Haustein UF. Anaphylactic shock and contact urticaria after patch test with professional allergens. Allergie Immunol 1976;22:349–52.

65. Maucher OM. Anaphylaktische Reaktionen beim Epicutantest. Hautarzt 1972;23:139–40.

66. Aalto-Korte K, Kuuliala O, Helaskoski E. Skin tests and specific IgE determinations in the diagnosis of contact urticaria and respiratory disease caused by low-molecular-weight chemicals. In: Giménez-arnau AM, Maibach H, editors. Contact urticaria syndrome. Boca Raton: CRC Press; 2015. p. 129–34.

67. Cromwell O, Pepys J, Parish WE, et al. Specific IgE antibodies to platinum salts in sensitized workers. Clin Allergy 1979;9:109.

68. Estlander T, Kanerva L, Tupasela O, et al. Immediate and delayed allergy to nickel with contact urticaria, rhinitis, asthma and contact dermatitis. Clin Exp Allergy 1993;23:306.

69. Lahti A. Non-immunologic contact urticaria. Acta Dermatol Venereol (Stockh) 1980;60(Suppl):3–49.

70. Clemmenson O, Hjorth N. Perioral contact urticaria from sorbic acid and benzoic acid in a salad dressing. Contact Dermatitis 1982;8:1–6.

71. Kligman AM. The spectrum of contact urticaria: wheals, erythema and pruritus. Dermatol clinic 1990;8:57–60.

72. Babilas P, Landthaler M, Szeimies RM. Anaphylactic reaction following hair bleaching. Hautarzt 2005;56:1152–5.

73. Barbaud A. Urticarires de contact. Ann Dermatol Venereol 2002;128:1161–5.

74. Von Krogh G, Maibach HI. Contact urticaria. In: Adam RM, editor. Occupational skin disease. New York: Grune & Stratton; 1983. p. 58–69.

75. Nicholson PJ. Evidence-based guidelines: occupational contact dermatitis and urticaria. Occup Medecine 2010;60:502–6.

76. Alfonso JH, Bauer A, Bensefa-Colas L, et al. Minimum standards on prevention, diagnosis and treatment of occupational and work-related skin diseases in Europe: position paper of the COST Action StanDerm (TD 1206). J Eur Acad Dermatol Venereol 2017;31(Suppl 4):31–43.

77. Zuberbier T, Asero R, Bindslev-Jensen C, et al. EAACI/GA$_2$LEN/EDF guideline: management of urticaria. Allergy 2009;64:1427–43.

# Protein Causes of Urticaria and Dermatitis

Alyssa Gwen Ashbaugh, MD[a,b], Mary Kathryn Abel, AB[a,c], Jenny E. Murase, MD[a,d],*

## KEYWORDS

- Protein contact dermatitis • Allergy • Cutaneous hypersensitivity reaction

## KEY POINTS

- Consider protein contact dermatitis when a patient presents with chronic, recurrent erythema, pruritus, burning, stinging and/or pain within a few minutes of contact with a protein allergen, particularly in a distribution reflective of a possible occupational exposure.
- Skin prick test is the gold standard for diagnosing protein contact dermatitis and is positive when a wheal at least 3mm greater in diameter than the negative control appears within 20 minutes.
- Allergen avoidance is the core of successful treatment and prevention of protein contact dermatitis, which may require personal protective equipment if the contact occurs in an occupational setting.

## INTRODUCTION

Protein contact dermatitis is a cutaneous hypersensitivity reaction to animal or plant protein.[1] Unlike the typical type IV hypersensitivity response to low-molecular-weight haptens that mediates allergic contact dermatitis,[2] protein contact dermatitis occurs in response to proteins of greater molecular weight.[1] In addition, protein contact dermatitis often causes an immediate wheal and flare response similar to contact urticaria and, in some cases, specific immunoglobulin E (IgE) antibodies to the proteinaceous material,[3] whereas allergic contact dermatitis causes a delayed hypersensitivity reaction.[2]

Conflicts of interest: Dr J.E. Murase has participated in Advisory Boards for Genzyme/Sanofi, Eli Lilly, Dermira, and UCB, participated in Disease Statement management talks for Regeneron and UCB, and provided dermatologic consulting services for UpToDate.

[a] Department of Dermatology, University of California, San Francisco, Third and Fourth Floors, 1701 Divisadero St, San Francisco, CA 94115, USA; [b] School of Medicine, University of California, Irvine, 1001 Health Sciences Rd, Irvine, CA 92617, USA; [c] School of Medicine, University of California, San Francisco, 533 Parnassus Ave, San Francisco, CA 94143, USA; [d] Department of Dermatology, Palo Alto Foundation Medical Group, 701 East El Camino Real (31-104), Mountain View, CA 94040, USA

* Corresponding author. Department of Dermatology, Palo Alto Foundation Medical Group, 701 East El Camino Real (31-104), Mountain View, CA 94040.

E-mail address: jemurase@gmail.com

Immunol Allergy Clin N Am 41 (2021) 481–491
https://doi.org/10.1016/j.iac.2021.04.008
0889-8561/21/© 2021 Elsevier Inc. All rights reserved.
immunology.theclinics.com

Protein contact dermatitis was first described in 1976 by Hjorth & Roed-Petersen in a study that analyzed the causes of occupational dermatoses in restaurant kitchen staff. They noted that although some food handlers experienced irritant dermatitis and/or contact dermatitis, another subset of kitchen staff experienced a distinctive, combined type I and type IV contact hypersensitivity reaction to proteins or proteinaceous materials.[4] Veien and colleagues further investigated this phenomenon and used a history of chronic, recurrent dermatitis caused by contact with proteinaceous material and a positive scratch test and/or radioallergosorbent test (RAST) as criteria to define protein contact dermatitis in their study population. In addition, it was noted that the reaction was marked by a burning sensation and pain rather than pruritus.[5] As described initially, protein contact dermatitis is predominantly observed in kitchen staff, as well as other occupations or hobbies that often come in contact with plant or animal proteins.[6]

This chapter reviews the epidemiology, pathogenesis, clinical features, common protein allergens, diagnostic process, treatment options, and prognosis of protein contact dermatitis.

## EPIDEMIOLOGY

Although the epidemiology of protein contact dermatitis has not been well characterized given the lack of formal, robust epidemiologic studies,[6] it has been reported to occur in 0.41% of patients with hand or forearm dermatitis[7] and 22% of patients with occupational skin disorders[8] in different geographic regions. Information from case reports and case series suggest that protein contact dermatitis predominantly affects chefs, caterers, dairy farmers, butchers, veterinarians, florists, and other workers who are frequently exposed to animal or plant proteins.[3] In addition, protein contact dermatitis to cosmetic products is becoming increasingly more common with the addition of natural ingredients to many cosmetics in recent years.[3]

Although there does not seem to be any increased risk between men and women for protein contact dermatitis, a history of atopy or chronic irritant dermatitis and occupations that result in chronic exposure to protein allergens have anecdotally been reported as risk factors for the development of protein contact dermatitis; this could be due to disrupted skin integrity, allowing for increased protein penetration,[9,10] or chronic skin irritation that induces a Th2-type response, promoting allergen sensitization.[11] Certain occupations have a predilection for protein contact dermatitis to specific types of allergens, which will be discussed further in the Common Protein Allergens section.

## PATHOGENESIS

The pathophysiological mechanisms underlying protein contact dermatitis are not well characterized.[12] Although many consider protein contact dermatitis to be a combined type I and type IV hypersensitivity reaction,[3] atopy patch,[13] skin prick, and scratch tests are typically positive in protein contact dermatitis, whereas patch tests are often negative on normal, noninflamed skin.[14]

There are 3 leading hypotheses regarding the pathogenesis of protein contact dermatitis. Many believe that protein contact dermatitis is elicited by a combined type I and type IV hypersensitivity reaction to a causal protein allergen. The type I quality of protein contact dermatitis is supported by the immediate urticarial type reaction observed in protein contact dermatitis that parallels the allergen-specific reaction observed in previously sensitized individuals. The type IV nature of protein contact dermatitis is reflected in the eczematous-like lesions associated with chronic exposure to the causative protein material and reports of delayed patch test positivity.[3,12] Patch tests are often negative in patients with protein contact dermatitis, and if the combined type I/IV theory is correct, this patch test trend is thought to be due to false-negative patch test results that may prove positive in the setting of occlusion or higher antigen concentration. Alternatively, negative patch test results could be explained by the fact that the protein antigens that cause protein contact dermatitis are too large to penetrate intact, normal skin. This justification is supported by the positive results yielded by skin prick or scratch tests, which break through the barrier of normal skin.[1]

Alternatively, a primary type I immediate hypersensitivity reaction with a superimposed allergic and/or irritant contact dermatitis has been proposed, given that protein contact dermatitis presents with wheals within minutes after contact with the causal protein, similar to a type I IgE-mediated hypersensitivity reaction.[3] In such a setting, the eczematous aspect of the dermatitis may in fact be more chronic in nature and secondary to a concomitant allergic or irritant contact dermatitis.[1]

Lastly, IgE-presenting Langerhans cells have been suggested as the drivers of IgE-mediated delayed hypersensitivity in protein contact dermatitis, similarly to their role in atopic dermatitis.[6] In atopic dermatitis, Langerhans cells bearing IgE receptors induce a delayed IgE-mediated reaction[3] and stimulate a Th2-type response.[11]

Histopathologically, protein contact dermatitis shares similarities with both allergic contact dermatitis and urticaria, demonstrating spongiosis with lymphocytic exocytosis and perivascular eosinophilic and lymphocytic infiltrates.[1]

## COMMON PROTEIN ALLERGENS

The proteins that cause protein contact dermatitis are divided into 4 groups: (1) fruits, vegetables, spices, plants, and woods; (2) animal proteins; (3) grains; and (4) enzymes (**Table 1**).[3] Naturally, different occupations have varying predilections for exposures to such protein allergens. For example, kitchen workers, caterers, food vendors/packers, and gardeners/florists are most likely to experience protein contact dermatitis from group 1 allergens, whereas chemical factory/pharmaceutical workers and detergent manufacturers are more likely to experience enzyme-associated protein contact dermatitis.[1]

Fruits, vegetables, and spices are group 1 allergens that commonly affect those who handle food, including gardeners, greenhouse staff, kitchen workers, and caterers. In addition, florists and plant researchers are commonly affected by group 1 allergens.[3] Very rarely, ingestion of raw fruit or vegetable allergens can result in dysphagia, tussis, dyspnea, rhinitis, or gastrointestinal symptoms.[1] Although natural rubber latex is a common cause of type I hypersensitivity reactions, it can also cause protein contact dermatitis in addition to allergic contact dermatitis and irritant contact dermatitis.[6,15] Given their frequent exposure to latex products, health care workers, veterinarians, and hair dresses were often affected by latex allergy[6] before extensive research and subsequent guidelines reducing its use.[3,12]

Although kitchen workers also often experience protein contact dermatitis to group 2 animal protein allergens, slaughterhouse workers, veterinarians, milk farmers, fisherman, and researchers who work with animals are similarly at risk for protein contact dermatitis mediated by group 2 allergens.[1,3,14] In addition, those who work with animal intestines are most susceptible, possibly due to the high protein–containing quality of such organs.[16] Interestingly, allergens that induce protein contact dermatitis are often species-specific and organ-specific, given that calf liver and chicken meat have been shown to induce a reaction, whereas chicken liver has not.[14]

**Table 1**
Four classifications and examples of protein contact dermatitis allergens

| Group 1 (First Half) | Group 1 (Second Half) | Group 2 | Group 3 | Group 4 |
|---|---|---|---|---|
| Almond | Horseradish | Amniotic fluid | Barley | Cellulase |
| Asparagus | Jalapeño | Amphibian serum | Chapatti | Chymotrypsin |
| Banana | Kiwi | Blood (cow, horse, lamb, pig) | Cornstarch | Glucoamylase |
| Bean | Lemon | Brains (cockroach, frog) | Gluten | Papain |
| Bishop's weed | Leek | Dairy products (cheese and milk [cow, dog, horse, and donkey]) | Oat | Protease |
| Cabbage | Lettuce | Dander/epithelium (cow, giraffe) | Rye | Trypsin |
| Cannabis sativa | Melon | Egg, yolk and white | Wheat | Xylanase |
| Caraway | Mushroom | Fishing fly | Chapati flour | α-amylase |
| Carrot | Natural rubber latex | Intestine (pig) | | |
| Castor bean | Olive | Hydrolyzed collagen | | |
| Cauliflower | Onion | Liver (calf/ox, chicken, lamb) | | |
| Celery | Orange | Locusts | | |
| Chamomile | Potato | Meat (cow, chicken, horse, lamb, pork, frog) | | |
| Chestnut | Paprika/pepper | Mesenteric fat (pig) | | |
| Chicory | Parsley | Parasites | | |
| Chives | Parsnip | Placenta (calf) | | |
| Chrysanthemum | Peach | Saliva (cow) | | |
| Coriander | Peanuts | Seafood/fish | | |
| Cotton | Pear | Seminal fluids (cow, dog, pig, human) | | |
| Cress | Pecan nuts | Silk | | |
| Cucumber | Pineapple | Skin/hair (cow, ferret, chicken, turkey) | | |
| Cumin | Potato | Suet | | |
| Curry | Rucola | Wool (ewe) | | |

| | | |
|---|---|---|
| Dill | Sapele wood | Worms/larvae |
| Eggplant | Sesame oil | |
| Endive | Spathe flowers | |
| Fig | Spinach | |
| Garlic | Tomato | |
| Gerbera | Walnut | |
| Green pepper | Watercress | |
| Hazelnut | Weeping fig | |
| Hedge mustard | Yucca | |
| Honey | Zucchini | |

Group 1: fruits, vegetables, spices, plants, and woods; Group 2: animal proteins; Group 3: grains; and Group 4: enzymes.
*Adapted from* Goossens A, Amaro C, Mahler V. Protein Contact Dermatitis. In: *Contact Dermatitis*. Cham: Springer International Publishing; 2019:1-10; with permission.

Not surprisingly, bakers are most commonly affected by group 3 flour allergens.[8] Patients with protein contact dermatitis to flour allergens are most likely to present with hand dermatitis; however, they can present with dermatitis of the forearms or face, or, uncommonly, a generalized distribution of dermatitis. In addition, asthma and rhinoconjunctivitis associated with protein contact dermatitis to group 3 allergens have been reported.[14]

Lastly, group 4 enzyme allergens most often cause protein contact dermatitis in pharmaceutical workers, factory workers, and detergent makers.[1] In addition, dough enhancer enzymes such as $\alpha$-amylase have been shown to induce reactions in bakers and are commonly associated with respiratory symptoms.[14] In fact, respiratory reactions are most common in group 4 enzyme-induced protein contact dermatitis compared with that induced by other types of allergens.[1]

In addition to the association of specific occupations with certain types of allergens, specific causes of protein contact dermatitis have been reported in greater frequency within distinct geographic regions, highlighting the influence of cultural customs on the development of protein contact dermatitis to particular allergens.[12]

## CLINICAL PRESENTATION

Protein contact dermatitis presents as a chronic, recurrent dermatitis that most commonly affects the hands and forearms in response to contact with a protein allergen.[1] Given that the lesions are confined to the areas of protein contact, different occupations often have varying distribution of involvement. For example, cases involving only certain fingers have been reported, most commonly in the setting of a chef cutting with their dominant hand and holding the food item with their nondominant hand.[4] Less common areas of involvement include the face[17] and proximal nail folds.[12]

Regardless of the distribution, protein contact dermatitis presents with erythema, pruritus, burning, stinging, and/or pain within a few minutes of contact with the causative protein allergen. Lesions may be vesicular, urticarial, or papular in nature.[1] Occasionally, extracutaneous manifestations, such as abdominal discomfort, diarrhea, and angioedema, may develop when the allergen is ingested.[14] In addition, asthma and rhinoconjunctivitis have been reported in patients with protein contact dermatitis after the ingestion of causal allergens.[7]

## DIAGNOSIS

Multiple laboratory tests can aid in the diagnosis of protein contact dermatitis, some of which are more informative than others. Importantly, if a patient has a history of systemic symptoms relating to the tested allergen, all diagnostic tests should be performed in an area with appropriate resuscitative facilities and trained medical professionals.[1,3]

Although there is scant literature on the sensitivity and specificity for skin prick testing for protein allergens in terms of diagnosing protein contact dermatitis, it is considered the gold standard diagnostic test for protein contact dermatitis.[3,7,18] Skin prick tests are widely used to assess sensitization to IgE and begin with the application of diluted test allergen, a positive control such as histamine dichloride, and negative control such as glycerinated saline histamine to the volar aspect of the forearm.[1,19,20] When positive, a wheal at least 3 mm greater in diameter than the negative control will appear within 20 minutes[18] due to the degranulation of mast cells in response to cytokines from the allergen.[20] Scratch testing works similarly but involves scratching the injected areas with needles. However, scratch testing is difficult to interpret and may have higher rates of false positivity compared with the skin prick test, thereby decreasing its sensitivity.[1,21]

Some investigators recommend performing an open application test, which involves rubbing the inciting agent on skin, before the prick and scratch test.[1,3] Although the open application test is noninvasive and inexpensive, it is typically negative unless performed on damaged skin.

The basophil activation test (BAT) has been discussed in the recent literature as a new diagnostic method for protein contact dermatitis.[3] The BAT is an assay that uses flow cytometry to measure the expression of activation markers on basophils, which are upregulated due to the presence of IgE antibodies.[22] Although this test has not been widely studied in the diagnosis of protein contact dermatitis and requires further investigation, it may be helpful in the identification of reactions to rare allergens.[3]

Other tests have been described in the literature regarding protein contact dermatitis but offer little diagnostic benefit. For example, the RAST measures the amount of allergen-bound IgE in serum but cannot evaluate tissue-bound IgE; as such, a negative RAST does not rule out a diagnosis of protein contact dermatitis.[1] Moreover, as stated earlier, there are several rare protein allergens that can cause protein contact dermatitis that would not be identified on RAST.[3] Histologic inspection of protein contact dermatitis will show nonspecific findings, including superficial perivascular lymphocytic infiltrate with eosinophils, spongiosis, acanthosis, and/or parakeratosis.[1,23] Histology is therefore often unnecessary for the diagnosis of protein contact dermatitis.

## DIFFERENTIAL DIAGNOSIS

There are several diagnoses that can mimic protein contact dermatitis, including allergic contact dermatitis, irritant contact dermatitis, contact urticaria, and atopic dermatitis.[1,24] To differentiate between these conditions, a thorough history, physical examination, and diagnostic work-up are essential. One of the key distinguishing factors of protein contact dermatitis noted throughout the literature is itching, burning, pricking, or pain that present immediately following contact with the inciting agent; however, large studies of patients with protein contact dermatitis indicate that this immediate reaction is only present between 7% and 15% of the time.[18,25] It is not uncommon for protein contact dermatitis to present with concomitant conditions such as allergic contact dermatitis or atopic dermatitis, making the diagnosis of protein contact dermatitis more complex and likely underreported.[1,3] As such, providers should remain suspicious of additional diagnoses if standard treatment methods for protein contact dermatitis are insufficient.

Both allergic and irritant contact dermatitis can mimic protein contact dermatitis. Allergic contact dermatitis is a type IV delayed-type hypersensitivity reaction caused by contact with a specific allergen and is a common cause of eczematous dermatitis. Although skin lesions may seem similar to protein contact dermatitis, patch testing will be positive, and skin prick, scratch, and RAST tests will be negative.[1,18] Irritant contact dermatitis, on the other hand, is an acute or chronic reaction to an exogenous substance that damages the epidermis of the skin. Irritant contact dermatitis can be differentiated from protein contact dermatitis primarily through history, as patients will often have a history of work, habits, or hobbies that can determine the possible causative exposure.

Protein contact dermatitis and contact urticaria due to proteins have long been reported together in the literature, further complicating the diagnostic picture.[7]

Together, protein contact dermatitis and contact urticaria encompass contact urticaria syndrome.[6] Contact urticaria will present with a wheal-and-flare reaction within 30 minutes following exposure to a protein that typically clears within hours without residual irritation but may result in generalized urticaria with angioedema or extracutaneous involvement.[6,24,26] Importantly, skin prick and scratch tests may be initially positive for patients with contact urticaria, but delayed reading will be negative.[1] Patch testing will also be negative in contact urticaria.

## TREATMENT

Allergen avoidance is the key to successful treatment and prevention of protein contact dermatitis. However, as noted by Levin and colleagues,[1] complete avoidance may not be feasible, particularly if the contact occurs in an occupational setting. Personal protective equipment such as gloves or protective clothing can assist in minimizing contact with the agents, as has been studied in chronic hand dermatitis.[27,28] Importantly, corn starch glove powder has been shown to be a cause of protein contact dermatitis, and prolonged occlusion with gloves may damage the dermal-epidermal layer and worsen protein contact dermatitis.[18]

If allergen avoidance is not feasible or sufficient, topical or systemic medications may provide moderate improvement, including topical corticosteroids, topical calcineurin inhibitors, and antihistamines.[1] However, as much of the literature on protein contact dermatitis comes from case reports rather than large, prospective studies, our understanding of the efficacy of these topical and systemic treatments is rather limited. Moreover, the efficacy of these medications may stem primarily from their treatment of concomitant conditions in protein contact dermatitis, such as atopic dermatitis or irritant contact dermatitis. High-potency corticosteroids can be used 1 to 2 times a day for limited periods of time to decrease inflammation, but must be expeditiously transitioned to low-potency to midpotency steroids or other alternative noncortisone topical medications due to the risk of atrophy with prolonged use.[1,18] Topical tacrolimus 0.1% and pimecrolimus cream 1% have been used in the treatment of chronic hand dermatitis and atopic dermatitis, and there are at least 2 cases documenting the use of tacrolimus in the treatment of protein contact dermatitis caused by chicken viscera and halibut.[1,29,30] Given the paucity of literature regarding the treatment of protein contact dermatitis, more research is needed to develop treatment guidelines.

## PROGNOSIS

Overall, the prognosis for protein contact dermatitis is favorable when allergen avoidance is used. Respiratory, gastrointestinal, ocular, or other systemic symptoms may occur if the inciting allergen is ingested.[7,18,31] Importantly, there are several reports that suggest significant personal and occupational consequences of protein contact dermatitis despite its favorable prognosis.[18,24,32] For example, Vester and colleagues[24] found that all individuals diagnosed with protein contact dermatitis in their study reported work-related consequences due to their condition, and these participants were more likely to have to change jobs, retire, or request sick leave than individuals diagnosed with other occupational food-related hand dermatoses such as irritant contact dermatitis or allergic contact dermatitis. Lodde and colleagues[32] posit that some individuals with protein contact dermatitis, particularly fisherman, may hide their condition out of fear of losing their jobs or having their medical clearance revoked. Thus, it is important for health care providers to recognize the burden of protein contact dermatitis and take steps to ensure that the treatment plan is aligned with the patient's needs.

## SUMMARY

Protein contact dermatitis is a cutaneous hypersensitivity reaction caused by chronic, recurrent exposure to animal or plant protein. Although protein contact dermatitis is known to predominantly affect chefs, caterers, dairy farmers, butchers, veterinarians, florists, and other workers who are frequently exposed to animal or plant proteins, epidemiologic data are limited and robust studies are warranted. In addition, although different theories regarding the pathogenesis of protein contact dermatitis exist, future studies are necessary to fully characterize the pathophysiological mechanisms responsible for protein contact dermatitis. With a more thorough understanding of disease pathogenesis, we will be better equipped to both diagnose and treat protein contact dermatitis in our patient population.

## CLINICS CARE POINTS

- Consider protein contact dermatitis when a patient presents with chronic, recurrent erythema, pruritus, burning, stinging, and/or pain within a few minutes of contact with a protein allergen, particularly in a distribution reflective of a possible occupational exposure.

- Skin prick test is the gold standard for diagnosing protein contact dermatitis and is positive when a wheal at least 3 mm greater in diameter than the negative control appears within 20 minutes.

- Allergen avoidance is the core of successful treatment and prevention of protein contact dermatitis, which may require personal protective equipment if the contact occurs in an occupational setting.

## DISCLOSURE

The authors have nothing to disclose.

## REFERENCES

1. Levin C, Warshaw E. Protein contact dermatitis: allergens, pathogenesis, and management. Dermatitis 2008;19(5):241–51.
2. Murphy PB, Atwater AR, Mueller M. Allergic Contact Dermatitis. In: StatPearls [Internet]. Treasure Island (FL): StatPearls Publishing; 2020.
3. Goossens A, Amaro C, Mahler V. Protein contact dermatitis. In: Contact dermatitis. Cham: Springer International Publishing; 2019. p. 1–10.
4. Hjorth N, Roed-Petersen J. Occupational protein contact dermatitis in food handlers. Contact Dermatitis 1976;2(1):28–42.
5. Veien NK, Hattel T, Justesen O, et al. Causes of eczema in the food industry. Derm Beruf Umwelt 1983;31(3):84–6.
6. Muttardi K, Kocatürk E. Immediate skin contact reactions induced by proteins. In: Giménez-Arnau AM, Maibach HI, editors. Contact urticaria syndrome: diagnosis and management. Switzerland: Springer; 2018. p. 75–89.
7. Barbaud A, Poreaux C, Penven E, et al. Occupational protein contact dermatitis. Eur J Dermatol 2015;25(6):527–34.
8. Vester L, Thyssen JP, Menné T, et al. Occupational food-related hand dermatoses seen over a 10-year period. Contact Dermatitis 2012;66(5):264–70.

9. Chen JK, Jacob SE, Nedorost ST, et al. A pragmatic approach to patch testing atopic dermatitis patients: clinical recommendations based on expert consensus opinion. Dermatitis 2016;27(4):186–92.

10. Gittler JK, Krueger JG, Guttman-Yassky E. Atopic dermatitis results in intrinsic barrier and immune abnormalities: Implications for contact dermatitis. J Allergy Clin Immunol 2013;131(2):300–13.

11. Thyssen JP, McFadden JP, Kimber I. The multiple factors affecting the association between atopic dermatitis and contact sensitization. Allergy Eur J Allergy Clin Immunol 2014;69(1):28–36.

12. Amaro C, Goossens A. Immunological occupational contact urticaria and contact dermatitis from proteins: a review. Contact Dermatitis 2008;58(2):67–75.

13. Walter A, Seegräber M, Wollenberg A. Food-related contact dermatitis, contact urticaria, and atopy patch test with food. Clin Rev Allergy Immunol 2019;56(1):19–31.

14. Janssens V, Morren M, Dooms-Goossens A, et al. Protein contact dermatitis: myth or reality? Br J Dermatol 1995;132(1):1–6.

15. Helaskoski E, Suojalehto H, Kuuliala O, et al. Occupational contact urticaria and protein contact dermatitis: causes and concomitant airway diseases. Contact Dermatitis 2017;77(6):390–6.

16. Hansen KS, Petersen HO. Protein contact dermatitis in slaughterhouse workers. Contact Dermatitis 1989;21(4):221–4.

17. Barata ARR, Conde-Salazar L. Protein contact dermatitis - Case report. An Bras Dermatol 2013;88(4):611–3.

18. Barbaud A. Mechanism and diagnosis of protein contact dermatitis. Curr Opin Allergy Clin Immunol 2020;20(2):117–21.

19. Pesonen M, Kallio MJT, Siimes MA, et al. Allergen skin prick testing in early childhood: Reproducibility and prediction of allergic symptoms into early adulthood. J Pediatr 2015;166(2):401–6.e1.

20. Birch K, Pearson-Shaver AL. Allergy testing. In: StatPearls. Treasure Island (FL): StatPearls Publishing; 2020.

21. Wakelin SH. Diagnostic methods: cutaneous provocation tests in contact urticaria syndrome. In: Giménez-Arnau AM, Maibach HI, editors. Contact urticaria syndrome: diagnosis and management. Switzerland: Springer; 2018. p. 123–30.

22. Hemmings O, Kwok M, McKendry R, et al. Basophil activation test: old and new applications in allergy. Curr Allergy Asthma Rep 2018;18(12):77.

23. So JK, Hamstra A, Calame A, et al. Another great imitator: allergic contact dermatitis differential diagnosis, clues to diagnosis, histopathology, and treatment. Curr Treat Options Allergy 2015;2(4):333–48.

24. Vester L, Thyssen JP, Menné T, et al. Consequences of occupational food-related hand dermatoses with a focus on protein contact dermatitis. Contact Dermatitis 2012;67(6):328–33.

25. Brancaccio RR, Alvarez MS. Contact allergy to food. Dermatol Ther 2004;17(4):302–13.

26. von Krogh G, Maibach HI. The contact urticaria syndrome—an updated review. J Am Acad Dermatol 1981;5(3):328–42.

27. Mygind K, Sell L, Flyvholm MA, et al. High-fat petrolatum-based moisturizers and prevention of work-related skin problems in wet-work occupations. Contact Dermatitis 2006;54(1):35–41.

28. Ramsing DW, Agner T. Effect of glove occlusion on human skin: (I). Short-term experimental exposure. Contact Dermatitis 1996;34(1):1–5.

29. Hordinsky M, Fleischer A, Rivers JK, et al. Efficacy and safety of pimecrolimus cream 1% in mild-to-moderate chronic hand dermatitis: a randomized, double-blind trial. Dermatology 2010;221(1):71–7.

30. Reitamo S, Wollenberg A, Schöpf E, et al. Safety and efficacy of 1 year of tacro-limus ointment monotherapy in adults with atopic dermatitis. Arch Dermatol 2000; 136(8):999–1006.

31. Kishimoto I, Kambe N, Nguyen CTH, et al. Protein contact dermatitis induced by cabbage with recurrent symptoms after oral intake. J Dermatol 2017;44(10): e252–3.

32. Loddé B, Cros P, Roguedas-Contios AM, et al. Occupational contact dermatitis from protein in sea products: who is the most affected, the fisherman or the chef? J Occup Med Toxicol 2017;12(1):1–6.

# Mimics of Dermatitis

Oksana A. Bailiff, MD, Christen M. Mowad, MD*

## KEYWORDS

- Atopic dermatitis (AD) • Allergic contact dermatitis (ACD) • Psoriasis
- Dermatophytosis • Scabies • Cutaneous T-cell lymphoma (CTCL)
- Subacute cutaneous lupus erythematosus (SCLE) • Dermatomyositis (DM)

## KEY POINTS

- The diagnosis of dermatitis can be challenging because many skin diseases can mimic dermatitis.
- It is important to recognize and be familiar with the skin diseases that can resemble dermatitis because some of them can represent signs of systemic disease, infection, infestation, or malignancies.
- Thorough history and physical examination, skin biopsy, and diagnostic tests are essential for establishing an accurate diagnosis and providing optimal care for the patient.

## INTRODUCTION

Dermatitis is a common condition frequently encountered by dermatologists. The diagnosis of dermatitis can be challenging because this condition is often multifactorial, and many skin diseases that can mimic dermatitis should be considered in the differential diagnosis.[1] When a patient presents with a pruritic, crusty, eczematous, and erythematous rash in a widespread distribution, clinicians most frequently consider the diagnosis of atopic dermatitis (AD) or allergic contact dermatitis (ACD), which are common conditions in dermatology. However, it is important to recognize and be familiar with other skin diseases that can resemble dermatitis but represent signs of systemic disease or malignancies because misdiagnosis can lead to mismanagement and adverse outcomes for the patient. What follows is a discussion of some of the diagnoses to consider when evaluating a patient with dermatitis.

## DERMATITIS ASSOCIATED WITH ALLERGY
### Atopic Dermatitis

AD is a chronic, pruritic, inflammatory skin condition characterized by a remitting and relapsing disease course.[2] AD occurs most frequently in children, with about 20% prevalence, and historically has been viewed as a pediatric disease, with 50% of

Geisinger Dermatology, 16 Woodbine Lane, Danville, PA 17822, USA
* Corresponding author.
E-mail address: cmowad@geisinger.edu

Immunol Allergy Clin N Am 41 (2021) 493–515
https://doi.org/10.1016/j.iac.2021.04.009
0889-8561/21/© 2021 Elsevier Inc. All rights reserved.

immunology.theclinics.com

atopic children developing this condition in the first year of life and 85% by 5 years of age.[3–6] However, AD is not only a disease of childhood but also affects many adults. It can persist into adulthood or present as adult-onset disease (**Fig. 1**A, B).[7] Prevalence of AD in adults in Western industrialized countries is reported to be around 5%.[8,9] This disorder is linked to many comorbidities and, in addition to other atopic march conditions, AD has been associated with increased reports of neuropsychiatric, behavioral, cardiovascular, and malignant diseases, suggesting that it should be regarded as systemic disorder.[10,11] The impact of the financial burden of this chronic condition on patients and society is substantial, with an estimated annual cost of $5.297 billion dollars in the United States in the year 2015.[12] The clinical presentation of AD varies with age and ethnicity.[3,13] Intensely pruritic, eczematous lesions accompanied by oozing, weeping, and crusting are common on the scalp, face, neck, trunk, and extensor extremities of infants, usually sparing the diaper area. In childhood, dry, erythematous scaly plaques are common in flexural sites such as the antecubital and popliteal fossa, neck creases, ventral wrists, and ankles.[2,8] Adults with AD have heterogenous clinical presentations, with higher prevalence of hand-and-foot dermatitis (**Fig. 2**A, B), nummular eczema, head-and-neck dermatitis, hyperlinear palms, erythroderma, generalized xerosis, lichenified skin changes, and prurigo nodules.[13,14] Because of diverse clinical presentations of adult AD, which differs from the classic flexural pattern of childhood disease, and lack of standardized diagnostic criteria, AD in adults should be regarded as a diagnosis of exclusion and other dermatologic conditions that can mimic AD should be carefully considered.[14] Adult-onset dermatitis may be over-diagnosed, and according to recent studies about 1 in 4 adults with AD self-report adult-onset disease.[3] The differential diagnosis of AD is extensive (**Table 1**) and includes inflammatory dermatoses, infestations, infections, immune-mediated conditions, and malignant diseases.[2,15,16] Good history, thorough physical examination, skin biopsy, and diagnostic tests are essential for establishing an accurate diagnosis and providing optimal care for the patient.

### Allergic Contact Dermatitis

A common differential diagnosis to AD is ACD.

ACD is an inflammatory skin condition caused by a delayed type IV hypersensitivity reaction in response to an allergen or allergens. The first step in the disease process is exposure to a chemical substance that results in a cascade of immune responses

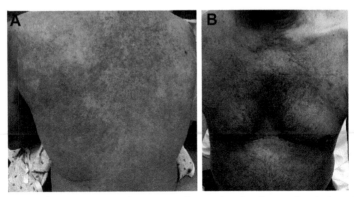

**Fig. 1.** (A, B) Adult-onset AD: erythematous, dry, and scaly plaques located on the back, chest, and abdomen of middle-aged white man.

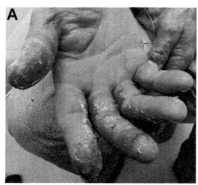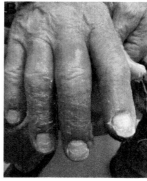

**Fig. 2.** (*A*, *B*) Hand dermatitis: erythema with scaling, crusting, and erosions involving the fingers and extending onto the palmar surface of hands.

resulting in sensitization. On repeat exposure in the sensitized individual, elicitation occurs with subsequent dermatitis.[17] ACD has a spectrum of clinical presentations. The acute phase is characterized by severe pruritus, poorly demarcated erythema, and edema expanding beyond the contact area as well as microvesiculations or, in severe cases, even bullae formation. In the subacute phase, scaly and crusty lesions develop with possible erosions. The chronic phase is characterized by less exudative lesions with features of lichenification, scaling, and fissuring.[17–19]

Acute ACD develops within 24 to 72 hours after allergen reexposure and initially presents with asymmetric eruption limited to the area of contact with the skin. However, it can soon become generalized, mimicking many dermatologic conditions, including AD and making diagnosis more challenging.[19] Therefore, the focus here is on differentiating clinical patterns of ACD from AD.

ACD presents on the face (including eyelids and perioral area), neck, hands, and feet; less frequently it can be seen on the trunk as a patchy generalized distribution and on the scalp. Patient populations at risk of ACD include those with occupational exposures, such as health care workers, beauticians, hair stylist, nail salon workers, auto mechanics, florists, construction workers, and industrial workers. Patch testing is a gold standard in the diagnosis of ACD.[20] Biopsy for histopathologic analysis to differentiate between ACD and AD is not helpful because both conditions look similar on hematoxylin-eosin and show spongiosis and superficial perivascular infiltrate with eosinophils.[17] Thus, clinical patterns, especially regional patterns, can provide a diagnostic clue and help distinguish ACD from AD and other dermatoses.

ACD of the face is most commonly caused by personal hygiene and cosmetic products (**Fig. 3**A–C).[21] Presence of eczematous plaques in the frontal hairline, on the sides of the face (sideburns) extending onto the lateral neck, and on the posterior neck can be consistent with allergens in hair dye, chemical perms, shampoos, or other hair products. The distribution of rash is caused by the product being applied to the scalp and subsequently rinsed off, leading to rash in the aforementioned distribution. The facial skin is more prone to ACD than skin of the scalp.[22]

Dermatitis of the central face presenting in bilateral patchy pattern can be caused by makeup, facial moisturizers, face washes, or gold being released from gold jewelry such as rings, watches, or bracelets reaching the face via the hands.[23] ACD of the eyelids is very common owing to frequent allergen exposure. However, as detailed previously, AD is also common in this location, as well as other skin conditions such as seborrheic dermatitis, psoriasis, and dermatomyositis (DM).[24] When eczematous

**Table 1**
**Mimics of dermatitis**

| Differential Diagnosis | Age of Onset | Distribution | Morphologic Features |
|---|---|---|---|
| Psoriasis | Children and adults. Bimodal age distribution in adulthood, with first peak around 20–30 y of age and second peak at 50–60 y of age | Classically: elbows, knees, extensor surfaces of the forearms and shins, umbilicus, intragluteal cleft, scalp, and nails. Other common locations: face (upper and lower forehead, periauricular area, ears, and cheeks), intertriginous/flexural areas, genitals, palms, soles, generalized (erythroderma) | Sharply demarcated oval, round, or irregular pink to erythematous plaques covered with thick, white to silvery scale. Lesions of psoriasis are dry, often causing fissuring and bleeding (Auspitz sign) |
| Dermatophyte infection | Children and adults | Scalp (tinea capitis), face (tinea faciei), beard area (tinea barbae), hands (tinea manuum), body (tinea corporis), groin (tinea cruris), feet (tinea pedis), and nails (tinea unguium) | Single or multiple red, annular or oval, scaly plaque varying in size with slightly raised active border and central clearing. Borders of the plaque have leading scale and advance centrifugally |
| Scabies | Children and adults | Infants and children: palms, soles, face, neck, and scalp. Adults: interdigital web spaces, flexural surfaces of the wrists, axillae, belt line, periumbilical skin, groin, buttocks, periareolar areas in women and penile shaft in men | Presence of burrows is pathognomonic, but can be difficult to detect because of secondary excoriations and crusting from frequent impetiginization. Intense nocturnal pruritus, urticarial papules, nodules, and vesicles represent the signs of host hypersensitivity reaction to the mite |
| Cutaneous T-cell lymphoma | Adults: between 50 and 60 y of age, M>F. Children: rare | Non-sun-exposed area or a bathing-suit distribution, which includes chest, lower trunk, buttocks, and groin | Classic morphologies are patch, plaque, and tumor stage. Early disease: well-defined, scaly erythematous patches or thin plaques with atrophic surface. Disease slowly progresses and can become widespread, and advanced stage characterized by infiltrative plaques, cutaneous tumors, erythroderma, and eventually nodal and visceral involvement |

| | | | |
|---|---|---|---|
| Subcutaneous cutaneous lupus erythematosus | Adults: between 20 and 40 y of age, F>M | Sun-exposed areas of lateral face, V area of the neck, upper back, shoulders, and extensor surfaces of the arms | Photodistributed, symmetric, nonscarring, erythematous macules and papules that evolve into either papulosquamous, psoriasiform plaques or scaly annular/polycyclic plaques with confluence, central hypopigmentation, and clearing |
| Dermatomyositis | Children: between 4 and 14 y of age<br>Adults: between 40 and 60 y of age, F>M | Gottron papules: dorsal surface of metacarpophalangeal and interphalangeal joints<br>Gottron sign: extensor tendons of dorsal hands in a linear fashion, dorsal-lateral sides of finger joints, elbows, knees, and medial malleoli<br>Heliotrope rash: periorbital, more pronounced on the upper eyelids<br>The shawl sign: posterior shoulders, upper back, and neck<br>The V sign: anterior neck and upper chest<br>The holster sign: lateral upper thighs and hips<br>Other areas: scalp, nailfolds, and hands (mechanic's hands) | Gottron papules: lichenoid, violaceous, flat-topped papules and thin plaques with slight atrophy and subtle scaling<br>Gottron sign: symmetric, slightly scaly erythematous to violaceous macules and patches<br>Heliotrope rash: symmetric periorbital violaceous erythema with edema<br>The shawl sign and the V sign: poikilodermatous skin changes (hypopigmentation or hyperpigmentation, telangiectasia, and atrophy) with macular violaceous erythema in photoexposed areas<br>Symmetric poikiloderma<br>Scalp: erythema, scale, and atrophy<br>Nailfolds: periungual erythema with telangiectasia of the proximal nail folds, dystrophic and ragged cuticles (Samitz sign), dilated capillary loops with dropout<br>Mechanic's hands: hyperkeratosis, scaling, and fissuring of the fingertips, palms, and lateral aspects of the first, second, and third digits |

*Abbreviations:* F, female; M, male.

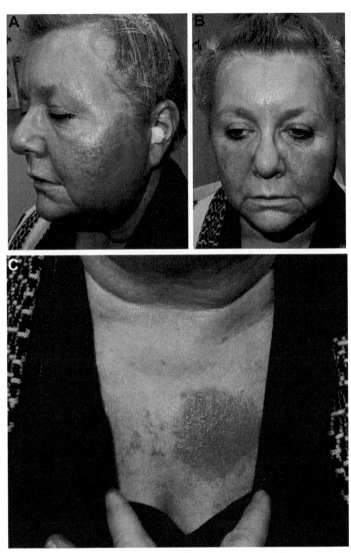

**Fig. 3.** (*A, B*) ACD of the face: erythematous, edematous plaque with small vesicles involving the face with sharp demarcation at the frontal hairline. (*C*) ACD to benzoyl peroxide.

plaques are located primarily on the lower eyelids extending down onto the cheeks in a linear, driplike pattern, eye drops should be suspected as a cause. Dermatitis involving both upper and lower eyelids in bilateral periorbital pattern can be caused by application of cosmetic products around the eyes. Importantly, an external allergen should be suspected when there is a unilateral eyelid dermatitis, which likely points toward transmission of an allergen from the hands.[22]

Dermatitis of the hands is very common. It is hard to differentiate chronic contact dermatitis of the hands based on morphology or histology from AD, dyshidrotic eczema, or palmoplantar nonpustular psoriasis.[25] Detailed history, including patient occupation and hobbies, followed by patch testing is extremely important if ACD is suspected. Dermatitis involving a tip of the thumb and the medial sides of the index finger and middle finger of the dominant hand in a pincer grasp pattern has been reported in florists from *Alstroemeria*, the Peruvian lily, *Chrysanthemum*, and *Hydrangea*.[22,26–28] Periungual eczematous dermatitis has been linked to nail cosmetics, specifically acrylates, and the number of cases have been increasing with increased use of photobonded acrylic gel nails.[29] Contact dermatitis from acrylic nails can also present on the face from airborne transfer of acrylic dust or direct transfer from the hands.

Foot dermatitis can result from the exposure to the allergens present in shoes, such as rubber, leather, and adhesives.[30] ACD of the foot can be mistaken for tinea pedis, psoriasis, dyshidrotic eczema, AD, and juvenile plantar dermatosis. Foot dermatitis caused by footwear usually occurs on the dorsum of the foot in bilateral distribution with sparing of the web spaces.[22] It is important to perform a scraping for potassium hydroxide (KOH) to rule out dermatophyte infection. If allergy is suspected, referral for patch testing is necessary.

## Psoriasis

Psoriasis is a common chronic, inflammatory, immune-mediated disease affecting about 2% to 3% of the general population.[31] Psoriasis affects both genders equally and can present at any age. However, bimodal age distribution is commonly observed, with the first peak around 20 to 30 years of age and a second peak at 50 to 60 years of age.[32] Psoriasis is a systemic inflammatory disorder and its involvement extends well beyond the skin. This condition is associated with multiple comorbidities, including psoriatic arthritis, cardiovascular disease, metabolic syndrome, gastrointestinal diseases, kidney disease, malignancy, and mood disorders.[33] It represents significant physical and socioeconomic burden and negatively affects quality of life in affected individuals.

Plaque psoriasis is the most common type.[34] It typically presents as sharply demarcated oval, round, or irregular pink to erythematous plaques covered with thick, white to silvery scale (**Fig. 4**). Lesions of psoriasis are dry, often causing fissuring and bleeding. They can cause pruritus as well as pain and burning sensation. Common locations include elbows, knees, extensor surfaces of the forearms (**Fig. 5**A, B) and shins, umbilicus, intragluteal cleft, and the scalp. Nail involvement is also common, affecting approximately 25% of patients with psoriasis.[34]

The differential diagnosis of psoriasis is vast and can include AD, nummular eczema, lichen simplex chronicus, pityriasis rosea, and tinea.[35] When clinical findings are distinctive with sharply demarcated, scaly erythematous plaques distributed symmetrically on extensor extremities, the diagnosis is straightforward. However, there are several variants of psoriasis, including atypical presentations that can mimic dermatitis and cause difficulty in diagnosis.

Facial psoriasis affects about 20% of patients with psoriasis vulgaris and is more commonly associated with longer disease duration and family history of psoriasis.[36] Clinical presentation is characterized by sharply demarcated, red, scaly, symmetric plaques associated with itching, soreness, and increased sensitivity. The most commonly involved areas of the face include upper forehead (76%), lower forehead (52%), periauricular area (46%), ears (39%), and cheeks (39%).[37] Psoriasis does not tend to affect eyelids, perioral area, or nasolabial folds.

Scalp psoriasis occurs in 45% to 56% of patients with psoriasis.[37] It can be easily confused with seborrheic dermatitis or tinea capitis. Lesions of scalp psoriasis are well-demarcated xerotic plaques with silvery-white flaky scale.[38] Plaques of scalp psoriasis are commonly located at the occiput and may advance beyond the border of the hairline. Affected areas of the scalp are extremely dry and are associated with cracking

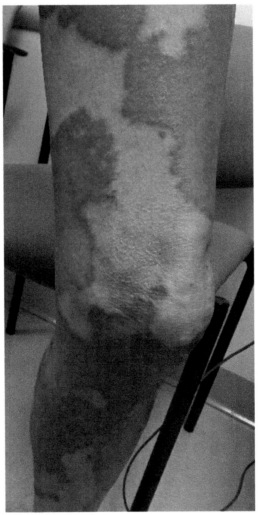

**Fig. 4.** Plaque psoriasis: sharply demarcated pink to erythematous plaques covered with scale.

and bleeding. Patients usually complain of pain, soreness, and burning sensation. Pruritus is a hallmark feature of scalp psoriasis that leads to scratching and picking.

Inverse psoriasis, also known as intertriginous or flexural psoriasis, affects 20% to 30% of patients with psoriasis. It involves the axillae, inguinal folds, intergluteal cleft,

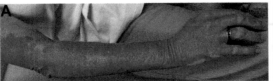
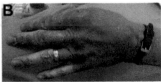

**Fig. 5.** (*A*, *B*) Psoriasis: sharply demarcated pink, scaly plaque involving the elbow, extensor surface of the forearm, and extending onto the dorsal hand and fingers.

neck folds, groin and external genitalia, umbilicus, postauricular area, and antecubital and popliteal fossae.[39] Skin lesions of inverse psoriasis are well-demarcated brightly erythematous smooth plaques that lack significant scale. They appear shiny and glazed because of the soft and moist flexural environment. Superficial erosion and maceration are common because of sweating and friction and can cause irritation and soreness.[38]

Palmoplantar psoriasis accounts for about 14% of cases.[34] This form of psoriasis is arguably one of the most debilitating and causes high morbidity and severe pain. It usually presents between 30 and 40 years of age and affects mostly women, with female/male ratio of 9:1.[40] Hyperkeratotic and pustular variants exist. The hyperkeratotic phenotype presents with red, dry, and thickened palms and soles with deep painful fissures.[36] The pustular variant presents with recurrent eruption of small sterile pustules and erythema on the palmar and plantar surfaces.[37] Diagnosis of palmoplantar psoriasis is challenging because of the clinical overlap with chronic ACD, dyshidrotic eczema, and AD with hand involvement.

Erythrodermic psoriasis is a very rare, potentially life-threatening form of psoriasis, affecting 1% of patients with psoriasis.[40] Erythroderma is an inflammatory skin syndrome that presents as generalized erythema and desquamation of more than 90% of the body surface area.[41] It is associated with high mortality because of loss of thermoregulation and skin barrier function that can lead to fever, hypothermia, fluid loss, electrolyte imbalance, dehydration, and shock.[40] Psoriasis is the most frequent cause of erythroderma, representing 25% to 50% of cases. However, other causes of generalized erythroderma include AD, drug reactions, cutaneous T-cell lymphoma (CTCL), pityriasis rubra pilaris, DM, Langerhans cell histiocytosis, and papuloerythroderma of Ofuji.[41] Distinguishing erythrodermic psoriasis from the other causes of erythroderma can be very challenging.

### Dermatophyte Infection

Dermatophytosis or tinea is a superficial fungal infection of the skin, hair, and nails caused by dermatophytes. Three major groups of dermatophytes that cause tinea are *Trichophyton*, *Epidermophyton*, and *Microsporum*.[42] Dermatophytes are the most common cause of superficial fungal infections in humans, with reported worldwide prevalence of 20% to 25%.[43] The most common sites of infection include the scalp (tinea capitis), face (tinea faciei), beard area (tinea barbae), hands (tinea manuum), body (tinea corporis), groin (tinea cruris), feet (tinea pedis), and nails (tinea unguium).[44]

Tinea corporis, colloquially known as body ringworm, involves the trunk, neck, arms, and legs. It classically presents as a red, annular or oval, scaly plaque, with slightly raised active border and central clearing. Borders of the plaque have leading scale and advance centrifugally. Lesions can be single or multiple and vary in size.[45] Tinea corporis can be easily misdiagnosed as nummular eczema, contact dermatitis or AD, seborrheic dermatitis, psoriasis, or erythema annulare centrifugum.[46] KOH 10% to 20% preparation applied to skin scrapings from the active margin of the lesion and examined under the microscope help establish the diagnosis of tinea. KOH scrapings are positive when refractile, long, smooth, branching, and septate hyphae are visualized (**Fig. 6**A–C).[42]

Tinea manuum is dermatophytosis of 1 or both hands and frequently occurs along with tinea pedis.[47] It presents as erythematous, dry and scaly, hyperkeratotic palms and is frequently confused with atopic hand dermatitis, irritant dermatitis, ACD, or palmar psoriasis.[48]

When cutaneous dermatophytosis is initially unrecognized, because of its resemblance to dermatitis, it is frequently treated with topical antiinflammatory agents

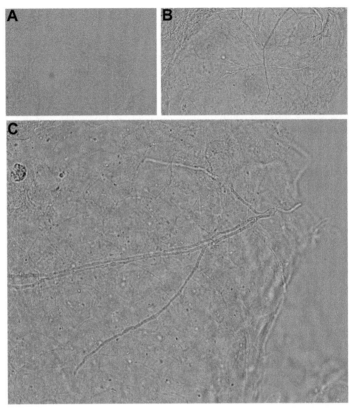

**Fig. 6.** (*A–C*) KOH 10% preparation positive for tinea with refractile, long, smooth, branching, and septate hyphae. (*A*) Original magnification x 200; (*B*) Original magnification x 400; (*C*) Original magnification x 400.

such as corticosteroids or calcineurin inhibitors. As a result, the dermatophyte infection loses its typical clinical and morphologic appearance, giving rise to an entity termed tinea incognito (**Fig. 7**A–C).[49]

Dermatophytosis can progress and become generalized, involving multiple body sites, including face, trunk, hands, and feet. When at least 4 body sites are affected, it is known as trichophyton rubrum syndrome.[50]

### Scabies

Scabies is a common, highly contagious, parasitic skin infection caused by the *Sarcoptes scabiei* mite. It is transmitted by close personal contact and indirectly via fomites. The estimated worldwide prevalence of scabies is 300 million cases every year.[51] In developed, industrialized countries, scabies is more frequently observed in the elderly residing in nursing home facilities, as well as in hospitals and overcrowded, impoverished areas. However, in developing countries, scabies is commonly diagnosed in children.[52] The diagnosis of scabies can be challenging because of the variety of clinical presentations. Scabies can mimic other skin conditions such as AD, allergic and irritant contact dermatitis, psoriasis, diaper dermatitis, drug eruption, and bullous pemphigoid.[53] Therefore, a high index of suspicion is needed to make a correct diagnosis. According to a recent study, approximately

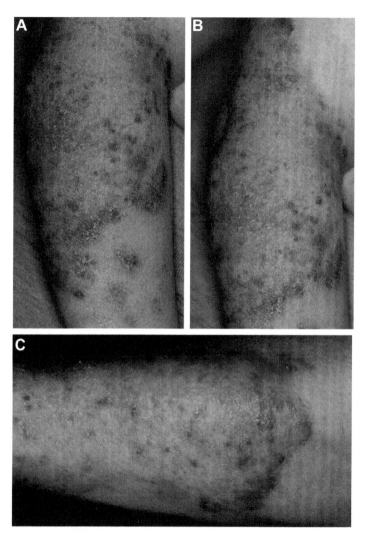

**Fig. 7.** (A–C) Tinea corporis treated with topical steroids (tinea incognito): erythematous, scaly plaques with partial central clearing and slightly raised active boarder with scattered papules and pustules.

45% of the patients presenting to the dermatology office with scabies had been misdiagnosed by another provider.[51,54]

Scabies infestation occurs when an adult female mite tunnels through the stratum corneum of the epidermis and lays 2 to 3 eggs daily. This activity results in a host hypersensitivity reaction to the mite invasion leading to signs and symptoms of infestation, including intense nocturnal pruritus, urticarial papules, nodules, and vesicles.[55] Detection of burrows is pathognomonic; however, it can be difficult because of secondary excoriations and crusting from frequent impetiginization.[56] In adults, common sites of burrows are interdigital web spaces, flexural surfaces of the wrists, axillae, belt line, periumbilical skin, groin, buttocks, periareolar areas in women, and penile shaft in men. In infants and young children, the palms, soles, face, neck, and scalp are frequently involved.[57]

The confirmation of the diagnosis can be made by obtaining a skin scraping of the burrow with a sterile #15 scalpel blade, placing the contents on a glass slide and applying a drop of mineral oil or 10% KOH preparation to the slide. Visualization of the mite, eggs, or mite's feces (scybala) under the microscope establishes the diagnosis. Because of the low sensitivity of this technique, it is strongly recommended to repeat the scraping in different areas.[58] Dermoscopy can be a useful tool for identification of the mite at the end of the burrow, which resembles a jetliner with contrail.[59]

Atypical clinical appearance, which further delays and complicates diagnosis of scabies, commonly occurs in patients on topical or systemic steroids (scabies incognito),[60] in immunocompromised patients with human immunodeficiency virus, as well as cognitively impaired elderly patients (crusted scabies)[61] and those with secondary bacterial infection and long-standing infestation where severe eczematous skin changes predominate.[62]

### Cutaneous T-cell Lymphoma

Mycosis fungoides (MF) and Sezary syndrome (SS) are the most common forms of CTCL, comprising more than half of the cases. The overall incidence of MF/SS is approximately 4 per 1 million people.[63] MF usually affects older patients between 50 and 60 years of age; however, it can be seen in younger patients, including children. Men are more commonly affected. MF is seen more frequently in African Americans compared with white people.[64] Patients diagnosed with CTCL have an increased risk of developing Hodgkin lymphoma and other nonhematologic malignancies.[65]

MF and SS are challenging to diagnose, especially in the early stages of the disease, because of numerous variants and clinical appearances mimicking many benign inflammatory dermatoses, such as eczema, psoriasis, nonspecific generalized dermatitis, and erythroderma.[65,66]

In classic MF, 3 clinical morphologies (patch, plaque, and tumor) are recognized **(Fig. 8A–C)**.[64] Early disease presents as well-defined, scaly, erythematous patches or thin plaques with atrophic surface in a non–sun-exposed area or a bathing-suit distribution, which includes the chest, lower trunk, buttocks, and groin.[65] Early-stage MF is indolent and very slowly progressive disease that can evolve over many years to decades to more widespread and advanced stages characterized by infiltrative plaques, cutaneous tumors, erythroderma, and eventually nodal and visceral involvement.[67]

MF is commonly referred to as a great imitator because of its wide clinicopathologic variants that mimic inflammatory conditions.[68] Such MF variants include, but are not limited to, hypopigmented, ichthyosiform, psoriasiform, and MF palmaris et plantaris, which contribute to the difficulty in diagnosing this disease.

Hypopigmented MF more commonly affects the pediatric population and skin of patients of color. It presents as round, oval, or irregular nonatrophic hypopigmented patches covered by fine scale.[69] Lesions are usually asymptomatic; however, sometimes they can be slightly pruritic. Hypopigmented lesions are typically distributed on the trunk, thighs, buttocks, and extremities.[70]

Ichthyosiform MF is characterized by widespread, dry, scaling patches and thin plaques with comedolike lesions and follicular keratotic papules involving the trunk and more commonly the extremities and resembling an ichthyosis vulgaris–like eruption.[69,71] This MF type is common in young patients and carries a relatively favorable prognosis.[72]

Psoriasiform MF presents with thick, scaly, well-demarcated, pink to erythematous psoriasiform plaques characteristic of psoriasis vulgaris. It is important to distinguish between these two conditions because systemic immunosuppressors used for treatment of psoriasis can exacerbate MF and possibly lead to accelerated progression of the disease.[71]

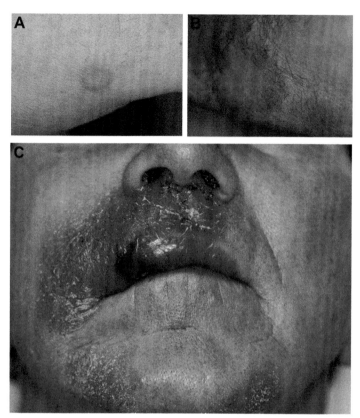

Fig. 8. (A) MF: thin, annular, eczematous plaque with erythematous boarder and atrophic center. (B) MF, plaque stage: annular, erythematous, alopecic plaque covered with fine scale on the forearm of white man. (C) MF, tumor stage: red-brown, eczematous, crusty, and scaly plaque with induration and nodularity involving upper vermilion and cutaneous lip of middle-aged white man.

MF palmaris et plantaris is a rare variant of MF that involves the palms and soles with occasional extension onto the dorsal aspect of feet, fingers, and wrists. Typical lesions are bilateral, annular, erythematous, hyperkeratotic, and sometimes hyperpigmented patches and plaques with fissures, scale, verrucous changes, ulcerations, and nail dystrophy.[69,71] Clinical differential diagnosis includes allergic and/or irritant contact dermatitis, dyshidrotic eczema, and palmoplantar psoriasis.[69]

SS is defined as an aggressive and leukemic variant of CTCL that is characterized by at least 1000 circulating atypical lymphocytes in the peripheral blood and erythroderma accompanied by severe generalized pruritus with or without lymphadenopathy.[63–66] Generalized exfoliative erythroderma can also present with keratoderma and fissures of the palms and soles.[65]

### Subacute Cutaneous Lupus Erythematosus

Subacute cutaneous lupus erythematosus (SCLE) is a subtype of cutaneous lupus erythematosus with distinct clinical presentation and serologic markers. Middle-aged women have much higher incidence of SCLE compared with men, typically with the disease onset in the third or fourth decade of life.[73] Approximately 25% to 30% of patients with SCLE are at risk of developing systemic lupus erythematosus; however, the systemic disease tends to be milder and is mostly limited to joint involvement.[74] Anti-Ro/SSA antibodies are detected in more than 70% of patients with SCLE and are the most common serologic association.[75] Secondary Sjögren syndrome is the most common autoimmune connective tissue disorder to overlap with SCLE.[76] SCLE is characterized by its high degree of photosensitivity, with ultraviolet (UV) light being one of the most common triggers.[75,77] Other environmental factors that can precipitate or worsen SCLE are cigarette smoking and certain medications, such as thiazide diuretics, calcium channel blockers, proton pump inhibitors, and allylamine antifungals.[78–80]

The skin lesions of SCLE are photodistributed, symmetric, nonscarring, erythematous macules and papules that evolve into either papulosquamous, psoriasiform plaques or scaly annular/polycyclic plaques with confluence, central hypopigmentation, and clearing (**Fig. 9**).[81] Sun-exposed areas of the lateral face, V area of the neck, upper back, shoulders, and extensor surfaces of the arms are frequently involved sites.[82] Clinically, SCLE eruption can be easily mistaken for annular lesions of psoriasis, tinea corporis, AD, nummular eczema, CTCL, or drug reaction.

Photoprovocation with UVA and/or UVB light can help confirm the diagnosis of SCLE. However, it might take up to 3 weeks for UV-induced eruption to occur.[76] Skin biopsy for histologic evaluation and direct immunofluorescence can also help support the diagnosis. Laboratory test for anti-Ro/SSA and anti-La/SSB antibodies should be performed. Previous studies showed that SCLE can present as paraneoplastic phenomenon associated with hematologic and solid organ malignancy.[74,83]

### Dermatomyositis

DM is a chronic, idiopathic, multisystem autoimmune condition that mainly affects skin and skeletal muscle. DM can occur in both children and adults. It has a bimodal age distribution, with 2 peaks occurring between 4 and 14 years of age (juvenile DM) and between 40 and 60 years of age (adult DM).[84] Similar to many other autoimmune diseases, DM has female predominance, with female/male ratio of 2:1, and it is more common in the African American patient population.[85] DM is further subdivided into classic DM, with both muscle and skin involvement; amyopathic DM (ADM), which includes pathognomonic skin rash of DM but lacks any clinical or laboratory evidence of

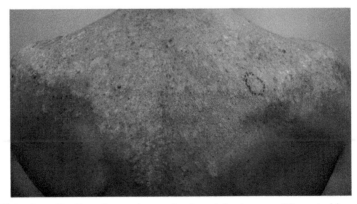

**Fig. 9.** SCLE: photodistributed, annular, coalescing pink plaques with central hypopigmentation located on the upper back.

myositis; and hypomyopathic DM (HDM), with subclinical muscle involvement and skin rash of DM.[86] DM is well known to be associated with an increased risk of malignancy, and some clinicians consider it a paraneoplastic phenomenon. Approximately 20% of patients with DM are diagnosed with solid organ cancers such as breast, ovarian, genitourinary, lung, and colon within the first 3 to 5 years after the diagnosis of DM is made.[87]

Cutaneous manifestations of DM can precede, parallel, or follow the onset of muscle disease. Amyopathic DM represents greater than 20% of all patients with DM.[88] A study showed that the risk of malignancy association for amyopathic DM is the same as for classic DM.[89] However, patients with some forms of amyopathic DM have a higher risk of developing a more severe form of interstitial lung disease that can be rapidly progressive and fatal.[90] Patients presenting without symptoms of muscle involvement can be easily misdiagnosed, which can lead to a lack of appropriate cancer screening and work-up for pulmonary disease.[88] Therefore, it is critical to recognize cutaneous features of DM and be able to distinguish this condition from other dermatoses that it can mimic, such as AD, ACD, seborrheic dermatitis, psoriasis, and cutaneous lupus.

The most common and pathognomonic skin lesions of DM are Gottron papules and Gottron sign. Gottron papules are lichenoid, violaceous, flat-topped papules and thin plaques with slight atrophy and subtle scaling overlying the dorsal surface of metacarpophalangeal and interphalangeal joints (**Fig. 10**).[84] Gottron sign represents symmetric, slightly scaly, erythematous to violaceous macules and patches overlying extensor tendons of dorsal hands in a linear fashion as well as the dorsal-lateral aspects of finger joints, elbows, knees, and medial malleoli.[86,87,90] Another hallmark cutaneous feature of DM is a heliotrope rash characterized by symmetric periorbital violaceous erythema that is more pronounced over the upper eyelids.[91]

Poikilodermatous skin changes with macular violaceous erythema in photoexposed areas of the posterior shoulders, upper back, and neck are referred to as the shawl sign. When these skin changes are present on the anterior neck and upper chest,

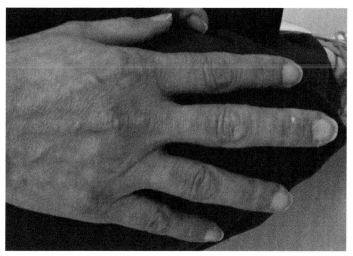

**Fig. 10.** Gottron papules: lichenoid, violaceous, flat-topped papules coalescing into thin plaques with slight atrophy and subtle scaling overlying the dorsal surface of the metacarpophalangeal and interphalangeal joints.

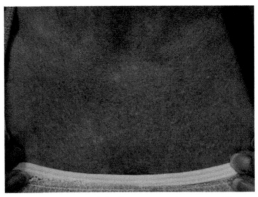

**Fig. 11.** V sign of dermatomyositis: poikilodermatous changes with macular violaceous erythema of the anterior neck and upper chest.

they are termed the V sign (**Fig. 11**). The presence of these lesions on the lateral upper thighs and hips is known as the holster sign.[90]

The involvement of the scalp in patients with DM is frequently accompanied by severe pruritus, which can be resistant to systemic treatment and can significantly affect the patient's quality of life.[92] Erythematous, scaly plaques of the scalp can look like ACD, seborrheic dermatitis, or psoriasis (**Fig. 12**).

Characteristic nailfold changes observed in DM include periungual erythema with telangiectasia of the proximal nail folds, dystrophic and ragged cuticles (Samitz sign), as well as dilated capillary loops with dropout (**Fig. 13**).[87,91,93]

Mechanic's hands is a known skin finding in DM that presents as hyperkeratosis, scaling, and fissuring of the fingertips, palms, and lateral aspects of the first, second, and third digits.[94] This cutaneous finding of DM is recognized as a clinical marker of the antisynthetase syndrome, which is associated with arthritis, Raynaud phenomenon, and interstitial pneumonitis.[93,95] Mechanic's hands of DM can closely mimic atopic, allergic, or irritant contact hand dermatitis and can easily be missed.

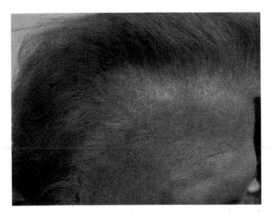

**Fig. 12.** Scalp involvement in patient with dermatomyositis: scaly, violaceous erythema of the superior forehead that extends into the frontal hairline.

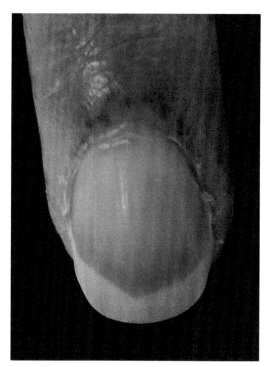

**Fig. 13.** Nailfold changes in dermatomyositis: ragged cuticle of the nailfold. Dilated capillary loops with dropout.

## CLINICS CARE POINTS

- Patients with AD are prone to ACD because of their epidermal barrier dysfunction. Therefore, AD and ACD can coexist in this patient population, which can make it even more difficult to differentiate between these two inflammatory skin conditions. Patch testing should be strongly considered in patients with AD in whom dermatitis is worsening, becoming more generalized, or is refractory to topical steroid therapy.[96]

- When facial psoriasis is suspected, examination of the patient's scalp is important because almost all patients with facial psoriasis also have scalp involvement.[36,37] Another diagnostic clue may be the presence of fine pinpoint bleeding after gently removing dry scale from the surface of the plaque, called the Auspitz sign.[40]

- Koebnerization phenomenon caused by injury and skin trauma results in worsening of the disease. Scalp psoriasis is vulnerable to koebnerization because of brushing, shampooing, scratching, and mechanical removal of thick scale by many patients who are unaware of this phenomenon.[36] History of disease exacerbation caused by trauma can provide a diagnostic clue.

- When considering a diagnosis of inverse psoriasis, asking the patient about genital involvement and performing a genital examination is of paramount importance because the groin is the most affected area in patients with inverse psoriasis, and external genitalia is involved in 80% of patients.[38,39]

- Checking for nail involvement, which is present in 25% of patients with psoriasis, may provide a diagnostic clue.[34] Look for irregular nail pitting, onycholysis, subungual hyperkeratosis, brown oil drop–like spots, nail bed discoloration, and splinter hemorrhages.[38]

- Most patients have a history of localized plaque psoriasis before the onset of generalized exfoliative dermatitis.[41] Therefore, obtaining personal and family history of psoriasis is crucial to establish a diagnosis. Other clinical clues include presence of palmoplantar keratoderma, nail changes, arthritis, and involvement of scalp, genitoanal, periumbilical, and retroauricular areas.[97]

- Two-feet-one-hand syndrome is a unilateral fungal infection of the hand that occurs with chronic bilateral tinea pedis.[98] Therefore, when diagnosis of tinea manuum is in question, it is prudent to check the patient's feet for tinea pedis.

- Secondary tinea usually results from autoinoculation of primary tinea pedis.[50] Check interdigital spaces of the feet for scale, maceration, fissuring, and peeling. Erythema, hyperkeratosis, and scaling of the sole, heel, and sides of the feet in a moccasin distribution can also be present.[47] Onychomycosis is common in chronic cases. Look for thickened nail plate with yellow discoloration, crumbling, ridging, and subungual debris.[99]

- Patient's history of intense pruritus that is worse at nighttime can provide a clue to the diagnosis of scabies.

- Scabies can occur in adults and children with preexisting eczema. Therefore, it is important to consider the diagnosis of scabies in any patient who presents with widespread dermatitis or pruritus of new onset, or with widespread impetigo.[100]

- Hypopigmented MF can closely resemble pityriasis alba, a cutaneous disorder that is common in children with AD. Pityriasis alba is found on the face, neck, and upper trunk, whereas, in hypopigmented MF, face and neck are usually spared.[70,101]

- Presence of alopecia, erosions, ulcerations, or indurated lesions can be clinical clues to the diagnosis on MF.[71]

- Diagnosis of MF palmaris et plantaris should be considered and ruled out in cases of long-standing hand-foot dermatitis that is poorly responsive to treatment or has atypical clinical presentation.[71]

- Erythroderma is an uncommon initial presentation of SS; therefore, in cases of nonerythrodermic dermatitis that is refractory to conventional therapy, diagnosis of early SS should be considered. Skin biopsy as well as testing for monoclonal T-cell receptor rearrangement and flow cytometry should be performed.[102,103]

- SCLE lesions can resolve with characteristic vitiligolike hypopigmentation or telangiectasia that subsides with time and does not lead to atrophy or scarring.[73,76]

- Heliotrope rash can be easily mistaken for AD or ACD of the eyelids. The important clinical feature that helps to make the correct diagnosis is the presence of periorbital edema, which always accompanies the heliotrope rash. The involvement of the orbicularis oculi muscle is responsible for the periorbital swelling and may result in the sensation of tightness and tenderness of the eyelids.[87,91]

- Unlike in hand dermatitis, pruritus is not a common feature of mechanic's hands. Also, patients usually deny any history of allergen exposure or the presence of preceding vesicular lesions. Resistance to topical ultrapotent corticosteroid therapy can be another clue to the diagnosis.[104]

## DISCLOSURE

The authors have nothing to disclose.

## REFERENCES

1. Nedorost S. A diagnostic checklist for generalized dermatitis. Clin Cosmet Investig Dermatol 2018;11:545–9.

2. Kapur S, Watson W, Carr S. Atopic dermatitis. Allergy Asthma Clin Immunol 2018;14(Suppl 2):52.

3. Lee HH, Patel KR, Singam V, et al. A systematic review and meta-analysis of the prevalence and phenotype of adult-onset atopic dermatitis. J Am Acad Dermatol 2019;80(6):1526–32.e7.

4. Nutten S. Atopic dermatitis: global epidemiology and risk factors. Ann Nutr Metab 2015;66(Suppl 1):8–16.

5. Hanifin JM, Reed ML. A population-based survey of eczema prevalence in the United States. Dermatitis 2007;18(2):82–91.

6. Silverberg NB. A practical overview of pediatric atopic dermatitis, part 1: epidemiology and pathogenesis. Cutis 2016;97(4):267–71.

7. Kim JP, Chao LX, Simpson EL, et al. Persistence of atopic dermatitis (AD): a systematic review and meta-analysis. J Am Acad Dermatol 2016;75(4):681–7.e11.

8. Simon D, Wollenberg A, Renz H, et al. Atopic dermatitis: collegium internationale allergologicum (CIA) update 2019. Int Arch Allergy Immunol 2019;178(3):207–18.

9. Barbarot S, Auziere S, Gadkari A, et al. Epidemiology of atopic dermatitis in adults: results from an international survey. Allergy 2018;73(6):1284–93.

10. Brunner PM, Silverberg JI, Guttman-yassky E, et al. Increasing comorbidities suggest that atopic dermatitis is a systemic disorder. J Invest Dermatol 2017;137(1):18–25.

11. Torres T, Ferreira EO, Gonçalo M, et al. Update on atopic dermatitis. Acta Med Port 2019;32(9):606–13.

12. Drucker AM, Wang AR, Li WQ, et al. The burden of atopic dermatitis: summary of a report for the national eczema association. J Invest Dermatol 2017;137(1):26–30.

13. Yew YW, Thyssen JP, Silverberg JI. A systematic review and meta-analysis of the regional and age-related differences in atopic dermatitis clinical characteristics. J Am Acad Dermatol 2019;80(2):390–401.

14. Silvestre salvador JF, Romero-pérez D, Encabo-durán B. Atopic dermatitis in adults: a diagnostic challenge. J Investig Allergol Clin Immunol 2017;27(2):78–88.

15. Barrett M, Luu M. Differential diagnosis of atopic dermatitis. Immunol Allergy Clin North Am 2017;37(1):11–34.

16. Siegfried EC, Hebert AA. Diagnosis of atopic dermatitis: mimics, overlaps, and complications. J Clin Med 2015;4(5):884–917.

17. Novak-bilić G, Vučić M, Japundžić I, et al. Irritant and allergic contact dermatitis - skin lesion characteristics. Acta Clin Croat 2018;57(4):713–20.

18. Johansen JD, Werfel T. Highlights in allergic contact dermatitis 2018/2019. Curr Opin Allergy Clin Immunol 2019;19(4):334–40.

19. So JK, Hamstra A, Calame A, et al. Another great imitator: allergic contact dermatitis differential diagnosis, clues to diagnosis, histopathology, and treatment. Curr Treat Options Allergy 2015;2(4):333–48.

20. Mowad CM, Anderson B, Scheinman P, et al. Allergic contact dermatitis: patient diagnosis and evaluation. J Am Acad Dermatol 2016;74(6):1029–40.

21. Mowad CM, Anderson B, Scheinman P, et al. Allergic contact dermatitis: patient management and education. J Am Acad Dermatol 2016;74(6):1043–54.

22. Rozas-muñoz E, Gamé D, Serra-baldrich E. Allergic contact dermatitis by anatomical regions: diagnostic clues. Actas Dermosifiliogr 2018;109(6):485–507.

23. Zirwas MJ. Contact dermatitis to cosmetics. Clin Rev Allergy Immunol 2019; 56(1):119–28.

24. Elmas ÖF, Akdeniz N, Atasoy M, et al. Contact dermatitis: a great imitator. Clin Dermatol 2020;38(2):176–92.

25. Kolesnik M, Franke I, Lux A, et al. Eczema in psoriatico: an important differential diagnosis between chronic allergic contact dermatitis and psoriasis in palmo-plantar localization. Acta Derm Venereol 2018;98(1):50–8.

26. Kamrani P, Nedorost S. The value of pantomiming for allergic contact dermatitis. J Am Acad Dermatol 2020;83(3):935–6.

27. Chu C, Marks JG, Flamm A. Occupational contact dermatitis: common occupational allergens. Dermatol Clin 2020;38(3):339–49.

28. Romita P, Ambrogio F, De prezzo S, et al. Occupational allergic contact dermatitis to Hydrangea spp. in an Italian florist. Contact Derm 2020;82(6):393–4.

29. Rieder EA, Tosti A. Cosmetically induced disorders of the nail with update on contemporary nail manicures. J Clin Aesthet Dermatol 2016;9(4):39–44.

30. Ortiz-salvador JM, Esteve-martínez A, García-rabasco A, et al. Dermatitis of the foot: epidemiologic and clinical features in 389 children. Pediatr Dermatol 2017; 34(5):535–9.

31. Michalek IM, Loring B, John SM. A systematic review of worldwide epidemiology of psoriasis. J Eur Acad Dermatol Venereol 2017;31(2):205–12.

32. Rachakonda TD, Schupp CW, Armstrong AW. Psoriasis prevalence among adults in the United States. J Am Acad Dermatol 2014;70(3):512–6.

33. Takeshita J, Grewal S, Langan SM, et al. Psoriasis and comorbid diseases: epidemiology. J Am Acad Dermatol 2017;76(3):377–90.

34. Merola JF, Li T, Li WQ, et al. Prevalence of psoriasis phenotypes among men and women in the USA. Clin Exp Dermatol 2016;41(5):486–9.

35. Tuzun B. The differential diagnosis of psoriasis vulgaris. Pigmentary Disord 2016;3(245):2376, 0427.

36. Aldredge LM, Higham RC. Manifestations and management of difficult-to-treat psoriasis. JDNA 2018;10:189–97.

37. Dopytalska K, Sobolewski P, Błaszczak A, et al. Psoriasis in special localizations. Reumatologia 2018;56(6):392–8.

38. Merola JF, Qureshi A, Husni ME. Underdiagnosed and undertreated psoriasis: nuances of treating psoriasis affecting the scalp, face, intertriginous areas, genitals, hands, feet, and nails. Dermatol Ther 2018;31(3):e12589.

39. Omland SH, Gniadecki R. Psoriasis inversa: a separate identity or a variant of psoriasis vulgaris? Clin Dermatol 2015;33(4):456–61.

40. Kimmel GW, Lebwohl M. Psoriasis: overview and diagnosis. Evidence-based psoriasis. Cham: Springer; 2018. p. 1–16.

41. Cuellar-barboza A, Ocampo-candiani J, Herz-ruelas ME. A practical approach to the diagnosis and treatment of adult erythroderma. Actas Dermosifiliogr 2018;109(9):777–90.

42. Sahoo AK, Mahajan R. Management of tinea corporis, tinea cruris, and tinea pedis: a comprehensive review. Indian Dermatol Online J 2016;7(2):77–86.

43. Kershenovich R, Sherman S, Reiter O, et al. A unique clinicopathological manifestation of fungal infection: a case series of deep dermatophytosis in immunosuppressed patients. Am J Clin Dermatol 2017;18(5):697–704.

44. Răducan ANCA, Constantin MM. To be or not to be tinea–Misdiagnosis and inappropriate treatment. Dermatovenerol (Buc) 2017;62:29–32.

45. Ely JW, Rosenfeld S, Seabury Stone M. Diagnosis and management of tinea infections. Am Fam Physician 2014;90(10):702–10.

46. Yee G, Al Aboud AM. Tinea corporis. In: StatPearls. Treasure Island (FL): Stat-Pearls Publishing; 2020.
47. Baumgardner DJ. Fungal infections from human and animal contact. J Patient Cent Res Rev 2017;4(2):78–89.
48. Chamorro MJ, House SA. Tinea manuum. StatPearls [Internet] 2020.
49. Maul JT, Maier PW, Anzengruber F, et al. A case of tinea incognita and differential diagnosis of figurate erythema. Med Mycol Case Rep 2017;18:8–11.
50. Nenoff P, Krüger C, Schaller J, et al. Mycology - an update part 2: dermatomycoses: clinical picture and diagnostics. J Dtsch Dermatol Ges 2014;12(9): 749–77.
51. Anderson KL, Strowd LC. Epidemiology, diagnosis, and treatment of scabies in a dermatology office. J Am Board Fam Med 2017;30(1):78–84.
52. Chosidow O. Scabies. N Engl J Med 2006;354(16):1718–27.
53. Arlian LG, Feldmeier H, Morgan MS. The potential for a blood test for scabies. PLoS Negl Trop Dis 2015;9(10):e0004188.
54. Stiff KM, Cohen PR. Scabies surrepticius: scabies masquerading as pityriasis rosea. Cureus 2017;9(12):e1961.
55. Chosidow O, Fuller LC. Scratching the itch: is scabies a truly neglected disease? Lancet Infect Dis 2017;17(12):1220-1221.
56. Engelman D, Fuller L, Steer AC. Consensus criteria for the diagnosis of scabies: a Delphi study of international experts. PLoS Negl Trop Dis 2018;12(5): e0006549.
57. Chandler DJ, Fuller LC. A review of scabies: an infestation more than skin deep. Dermatology (Basel) 2019;235(2):79–90.
58. Micali G, Lacarrubba F, Verzì AE, et al. Scabies: advances in noninvasive diagnosis. PLoS Negl Trop Dis 2016;10(6):e0004691.
59. Park JH, Kim CW, Kim SS. The diagnostic accuracy of dermoscopy for scabies. Ann Dermatol 2012;24(2):194–9.
60. Kim KJ, Roh KH, Choi JH, et al. Scabies incognito presenting as urticaria pigmentosa in an infant. Pediatr Dermatol 2002;19(5):409–11.
61. Raffi J, Suresh R, Butler DC. Review of Scabies in the Elderly. Dermatol Ther (Heidelb) 2019;9(4):623–30.
62. McCarthy JS, Kemp DJ, Walton SF, et al. Scabies: more than just an irritation. Postgrad Med J 2004;80(945):382–7.
63. Foss FM, Girardi M. Mycosis fungoides and sezary syndrome. Hematol Oncol Clin North Am 2017;31(2):297–315.
64. Larocca C, Kupper T. Mycosis fungoides and Sézary syndrome: an update. Hematology/Oncology Clin 2019;33(1):103–20.
65. Jawed SI, Myskowski PL, Horwitz S, et al. Primary cutaneous T-cell lymphoma (mycosis fungoides and Sezary syndrome): part I. Diagnosis: clinical and histo-pathologic features and new molecular and biologic markers. J Am Acad Dermatol 2014;70(2):205.
66. Wilcox RA. Cutaneous T-cell lymphoma: 2016 Update on diagnosis, risk-stratification, and management. Am J Hematol 2016;91(1):152–65.
67. Scarisbrick JJ, Quaglino P, Prince HM, et al. The PROCLIPI international registry of early stage mycosis fungoides identifies substantial diagnostic delay in most patients. Br J Dermatol 2019;181(2):350–7.
68. Kelati A, Gallouj S, Tahiri L, et al. Defining the mimics and clinico-histological diagnosis criteria for mycosis fungoides to minimize misdiagnosis. Int J Womens Dermatol 2017;3(2):100–6.

69. Ahn CS, ALSayyah A, Sangüeza OP. Mycosis fungoides: an updated review of clinicopathologic variants. Am J Dermatopathol 2014;36:933–48.

70. Rodney IJ, Kindred C, Angra K, et al. Hypopigmented mycosis fungoides: a retrospective clinicohistopathologic study. J Eur Acad Dermatol Venereol 2017;31:808–14.

71. Hodak E, Amitay-Iaish I. Mycosis fungoides: A great imitator. Clin Dermatol 2019;37(3):255–67.

72. Jang MS, Kang DY, Park JB, et al. Clinicopathological manifestations of ichthyosiform mycosis fungoides. Acta Derm Venereol 2016;96:100–1.

73. Jatwani S, Hearth Holmes MP. Subacute cutaneous lupus erythematosus. In: StatPearls. Treasure Island (FL): StatPearls Publishing; 2020.

74. Blake SC, Daniel BS. Cutaneous lupus erythematosus: a review of the literature. Int J Womens Dermatol 2019;5(5):320–9.

75. Achtman JC, Werth VP. Pathophysiology of cutaneous lupus erythematosus. Arthritis Res Ther 2015;17:182.

76. Szczęch J, Rutka M, Samotij D, et al. Clinical characteristics of cutaneous lupus erythematosus. Postepy Dermatol Alergol 2016;33(1):13–7.

77. Kuhn A, Ruland V, Bonsmann G. Photosensitivity, phototesting, and photoprotection in cutaneous lupus erythematosus. Lupus 2010;19(9):1036–46.

78. Little AJ, Vesely MD. Cutaneous lupus erythematosus: current and future pathogenesis-directed therapies. Yale J Biol Med 2020;93(1):81–95.

79. Lowe GC, Lowe G, Henderson CL, et al. A systematic review of drug-induced subacute cutaneous lupus erythematosus. Br J Dermatol 2011;164(3):465–72.

80. Jarrett P, Werth VP. A review of cutaneous lupus erythematosus: improving outcomes with a multidisciplinary approach. J Multidiscip Healthc 2019;12:419–28.

81. Kuhn A, Landmann A. The classification and diagnosis of cutaneous lupus erythematosus. J Autoimmun 2014;48-49:14–9.

82. Alniemi DT, Gutierrez A Jr, Drage LA, et al. Subacute cutaneous lupus erythematosus: clinical characteristics, disease associations, treatments, and outcomes in a series of 90 patients at mayo clinic, 1996-2011. Mayo Clin Proc 2017; 92(3):406–14.

83. Evans KG, Heymann WR. Paraneoplastic subacute cutaneous lupus erythematosus: an underrecognized entity. Cutis 2013;91(1):25–9.

84. Dewane ME, Waldman R, Lu J. Dermatomyositis: clinical features and pathogenesis. J Am Acad Dermatol 2020;82(2):267–81.

85. Chansky PB, Olazagasti JM, Feng R, et al. Cutaneous dermatomyositis disease course followed over time using the cutaneous dermatomyositis disease area and severity index. J Am Acad Dermatol 2018;79(3):464–9.e2.

86. Iaccarino L, Ghirardello A, Bettio S, et al. The clinical features, diagnosis and classification of dermatomyositis. J Autoimmun 2014;48-49:122–7.

87. Bogdanov I, Kazandjieva J, Darlenski R, et al. Dermatomyositis: Current concepts. Clin Dermatol 2018;36(4):450–8.

88. Patel B, Khan N, Werth VP. Applicability of EULAR/ACR classification criteria for dermatomyositis to amyopathic disease. J Am Acad Dermatol 2018;79(1): 77–83.e1.

89. El-azhary RA, Pakzad SY. Amyopathic dermatomyositis: retrospective review of 37 cases. J Am Acad Dermatol 2002;46(4):560–5.

90. Mainetti C, Beretta-Piccoli BT, Selmi C. Cutaneous manifestations of dermatomyositis: a comprehensive review. Clin Rev Allergy Immunol 2017;53(3):337–56.

91. Santmyire-rosenberger B, Dugan EM. Skin involvement in dermatomyositis. Curr Opin Rheumatol 2003;15(6):714–22.

92. Hundley JL, Carroll CL, Lang W, et al. Cutaneous symptoms of dermatomyositis significantly impact patients' quality of life. J Am Acad Dermatol 2006;54(2): 217–20.

93. Sontheimer RD. Dermatomyositis: an overview of recent progress with emphasis on dermatologic aspects. Dermatol Clin 2002;20(3):387-408.

94. Wernham M, Montague SJ. Mechanic's hands and hiker's feet in antisynthetase syndrome. CMAJ 2017;189(44):E1365.

95. Cox JT, Gullotti DM, Mecoli CA, et al. "Hiker's feet": a novel cutaneous finding in the inflammatory myopathies. Clin Rheumatol 2017;36(7):1683–6.

96. Owen JL, Vakharia PP, Silverberg JI. The role and diagnosis of allergic contact dermatitis in patients with atopic dermatitis. Am J Clin Dermatol 2018;19(3): 293–302.

97. Boehncke WH, Schön MP. Psoriasis. Lancet 2015;386(9997):983–94.

98. Singri P, Brodell RT. 'Two feet-one hand' syndrome: a recurring infection with a peculiar connection. Postgrad Med 1999;106(2):83–4.

99. Lipner SR, Scher RK. Onychomycosis: clinical overview and diagnosis. J Am Acad Dermatol 2019;80(4):835–51.

100. Johnston G, Sladden M. Scabies: diagnosis and treatment. BMJ 2005; 331(7517):619–22.

101. Amorim GM, Niemeyer-Corbellini JP, Quintella DC, et al. Hypopigmented mycosis fungoides: a 20-case retrospective series. Int J Dermatol 2018;57: 306–12.

102. Mangold AR, Thompson Ak, Davis MD, et al. Early clinical manifestations of Sezary syndrome: a multicenter retrospective cohort study. J Am Acad Dermatol 2017;77(4):719–27.

103. Thompson AK, Killian JM, Weaver AL, et al. Sézary syndrome without erythroderma: a review of 16 cases at Mayo Clinic. J Am Acad Dermatol 2017;76(4): 683–8.

104. Concha JSS, Merola JF, Fiorentino D, et al. Re-examining mechanic's hands as a characteristic skin finding in dermatomyositis. J Am Acad Dermatol 2018;78(4): 769–75.e2.

# Food Allergy Evaluation for Dermatologic Disorders

Kanwaljit K. Brar, MD[a,b]

## KEYWORDS

- Food allergy • Atopic dermatitis • Contact urticaria • Protein contact dermatitis
- Early food introduction

## KEY POINTS

- Specific Immunoglobulin E (IgE) testing and skin prick testing can be used to identify the causative allergen in contact urticaria and protein contact dermatitis; fresh food testing carries a risk of systemic reaction.
- Infants with atopic dermatitis are at increased risk for development of life-threatening food allergy, and their risk increases with increasing severity of dermatitis.
- Clinicians should advise infants with mild-to-moderate atopic dermatitis of early introduction of allergenic foods as early as 6 months of life.
- Clinical relevance of positive food allergy tests should be determined by the allergist and may warrant performance of oral food challenge, the definitive test for diagnosis of IgE-mediated food allergy.

## BACKGROUND

When evaluating dermatitis, clinicians are often presented with patients inquiring about the relationship of their rash to food allergy. Food allergy refers to the breakdown of clinical and immune tolerance to ingested foods. Food allergy may be immunoglobulin E (IgE) mediated, as in food-induced anaphylaxis, or non-IgE mediated, as in food protein–induced allergic proctocolitis, food protein–induced enterocolitis syndrome or eosinophilic esophagitis. IgE-mediated food allergy is defined by the presence of one or more immediate symptoms within 2 hours of ingestion of a food. Symptoms may be mild, and cutaneous only with hives or erythema, or more severe, resulting in 2-system involvement, such as angioedema, difficulty breathing, pharyngeal edema, vomiting, and hemodynamic instability, which can be life-threatening. The development of IgE-mediated food allergy is related to underlying atopy, or predisposition toward allergy, which can be attributed to an upregulated type II immune system often brought on by atopic dermatitis (AD), known as the atopic march.

[a] Fink Pediatric Ambulatory Care Center 160 East 32nd St, 3rd floor New York, NY 10016, USA;
[b] Department of Pediatrics, NYU Grossman School of Medicine, Hassenfeld Children's Hospital, 160 East 32nd Street, L3, New York, NY 10016, USA
E-mail address: kanwaljit.brar@nyulangone.org

Immunol Allergy Clin N Am 41 (2021) 517–526
https://doi.org/10.1016/j.iac.2021.04.010
0889-8561/21/© 2021 Elsevier Inc. All rights reserved.
immunology.theclinics.com

AD is a complex, multifactorial disease related to immune and barrier dysregulation that remits and relapses often without a clearly identifiable trigger. In one study in Europe, children with AD undergoing double-blind placebo-controlled food challenges for suspected food allergies experienced higher positive reaction rates with increasingly severe AD. Children with mild, moderate, and severe AD had positive reaction rates of 53.3%, 51.7%, and 100%, respectively.[1] These findings support the hypothesis that children with more severe AD are at higher risk for immediate food allergy.[1] Patients with mild AD are often not considered to be at increased risk for food allergy; however, the DBPC findings demonstrate that even patients with mild AD have similar reaction rates to foods as patients with more severe AD.

The top allergens causing 90% of food allergies in children with AD are cow's milk, hen's egg, peanut, wheat, soy, tree nuts, and fish.[2] In older children and adults, birch-pollen related foods, such as fruits and vegetables in the *Rosaceae, Umbelliferae,* and *Solanaceae* families can cause delayed AD exacerbations, although these are not the typical oral IgE-mediated symptoms experienced with raw foods in oral allergy syndrome.[2] Food-related AD exacerbations are mixed mechanism, and some studies have demonstrated benefit of elimination diets, for example, exclusion of hen's egg and milk to treat AD. However, these diets may harm patients nutritionally, removing important sources of macronutrients and micronutrients from the diet, which can be detrimental to a growing child. Atopy patch tests have been used to identify causative foods of AD exacerbation, but testing is not standardized and has not been recommended in any formal guidelines for management of AD.[2] Thus, foods have an unclear role in triggering AD exacerbations, but there is a clear association for a comorbidity of food allergy in AD. Infants with features of chronic eczema or who meet criteria for severe AD should be considered for allergy referral to screen for food allergies to the highly allergenic foods, as these may pose a risk when newly introduced. Here, the authors review food allergy evaluation for dermatologic disorders and summarize reasons for an allergist's referral in **Box 1**.

## MECHANISM

Mechanisms of predisposition toward food allergy may be tied to immune programming and barrier abnormalities inherent to the skin of individuals with AD[3]; this has

---

**Box 1**
**Reasons for allergist referral in dermatologic disorders**

- Presence of allergic disorders such as allergic rhinitis, asthma, food allergy, oral allergy syndrome, etc.
- Performance of skin prick testing to identify comorbidities and suspected food or environmental triggers for contact urticaria, protein contact dermatitis, and/or atopic dermatitis
- Any clinical history of immediate or delayed food allergic reaction including hives, gastrointestinal, respiratory, throat symptoms, or hemodynamic instability
- Any positive food-specific IgE tests (>0.35 kU/L)
- Performance of oral food challenge (OFC)
- Consider in infants at high risk for development of food allergy (severe AD)
- Family reluctance to introduce foods and desire for monitored food introductions

been demonstrated by Kim and colleagues in human and mouse models of AD, which show clusters of basophils and type II innate lymphoid cells in inflamed skin.[3] These cells can release the type II cytokine interleukin-4 (IL-4), which can further promote T-cell differentiation into Th2 helper cells, and promote release of additional type II cytokines, such as IL-4, IL-5, IL-13, and IL-31. Emerging evidence shows that even in nonlesional skin of patients with AD and food allergy, there are abnormalities in lipid composition and filaggrin expression.[4] Mice and human models further prove that food protein exposures via nonlesional skin may result in sensitization and clinical food allergy.[4,5] The occurrence of this cutaneous sensitization may be mediated by epithelial-derived cytokines, such as IL-25, IL-33, and thymic stromal lymphopoietin.[6] These skin abnormalities may manifest clinically with physical examination findings, such as hyperlinear palms, which have recently been associated with sensitization to hen's egg and peanut allergy.[7,8]

## PROTEIN CONTACT DERMATITIS

Food protein contact dermatitis represent an entity with features of type I IgE-mediated food allergy and type IV T cell–mediated dermatitis.[9] Individuals typically present with hand eczema or food protein–induced contact urticaria (CU). Characteristic rash can present with immediate erythema and pruritus that may later develop into a vesicular rash, and individuals may also develop paronychial inflammation. Food protein contact dermatitis typically occurs in food handlers with occupational exposures to food proteins, such as cooks and bakers, who are exposed to proteins in foods, such as fish and wheat.[9] Confirmatory diagnosis is made via skin prick testing (SPT), as the mechanism is thought to be IgE mediated. Patch tests are often negative.

In a retrospective analysis of 7560 patients in a French Dermatology and Allergy clinic, 31 patients with PCD were identified, of which 22 patients had occupational exposures.[9] Of the 22 occupationally related cases, 18 occurred in food handlers and 12 occurred in cooks, of which 5 were sensitized to fish, 2 to shellfish, 2 to meat, 2 to nuts, and 1 to multiple foods.[9] Six cases occurred in other food handlers, including 3 bakers who were all sensitized to flour and 1 baker who was sensitized to nuts.[9] Among this smaller cohort, approximately two-thirds (68%) had associated atopy.[9] Similarly, in another European study of 291 cases of PCD and CU, almost half had associated respiratory disease, which in 21% of those with occupational asthma and 38% of those with occupational rhinitis was caused by the same allergen causing the skin findings.[10] Interestingly, as children with atopic dermatitis who undergo immune transformation, that is, the atopic march, a small population of patients with food PCD are also at risk for future anaphylaxis. Their background history of atopy may set up an immune predisposition to cutaneous sensitization, much as the infant with atopic dermatitis, and similarly, both populations warrant an allergist's referral.

## DIAGNOSIS

For the diagnosis of protein CU, SPT is the preferred test. SPT may be conducted using 2 modalities, commercial extracts, or prick-to-prick (PTP) tests in which the food is pricked and then the patient's skin is pricked. Pricking is accomplished with the use of a hypodermic needle, or lancet, which is typically plastic, although sometimes has a metal tip, and is used to prick the epidermal skin surface with allergen.[11] Tests are performed on the volar forearm or upper back. Allergen exposure results in cross-linking of IgE on the mast cell surface, which results in the release of histamine, and subsequent wheal and flare reaction. Interpretation of the test should be done after 15 minutes and involves measurement of the mean wheal diameter and erythema (flare) at each individual prick site.[12] A glycerinated saline solution and histamine (10 mg/mL) solution are used as negative and positive control, respectively, and allow for test validation. Pricks are placed 2 cm apart to avoid overlapping wheal and flare reactions.[12] Tests are considered positive if they are 3 mm greater than the negative control, or equal to, or larger than the histamine control. Antihistamines must be discontinued 5 to 7 days before anticipated SPT, as recent antihistamine use will interfere with the histamine response being measured. Stopping antihistamines can create difficulties in the urticaria patient relying on daily antihistamine therapy, and patients should counseled as such before scheduling an SPT visit.

Pricking with commercial extracts is the preferred method for diagnosis of typical IgE-mediated food allergy against the most common allergenic foods, that is, cow's-milk, peanut, tree nuts, hen's egg, wheat, and soy. PTP testing is the preferred method for testing in oral allergy syndrome, which is the presence of oral itching, tingling, and sometimes swelling with consumption of fruits and vegetables due to cross-reactivities with pollens. Because symptoms are typically due to fresh fruits and vegetables, pricking with commercial extracts is less sensitive.[11] PTP testing may also be useful when testing for allergy to fish or shellfish.[11–13] PTP testing can raise issues of which portion of the food is most appropriate to use for testing. For example, with apple there is a statistically significant difference in prick tests obtained from material near the stalk of the apple, compared with the middle of the apple, with tests near the stalk yielding more positive results.[14] The same is true for other fruits, such as citrus fruits, where the peel, pulp, and seeds may contain different allergens.[15] In peaches, the allergens from the peel can result in anaphylaxis in the same patient who may tolerate ingesting the peeled fruit.[16] In such situations where skin testing results may vary based on method, confirmatory diagnosis of the relevant allergen may be better delineated using serum IgE testing with component resolved diagnostics. For example, for peach, allergy to the lipid transfer protein Pru p3 is more common, whereas allergy to Pru p7, a gibberellin-regulated protein, is associated with severe anaphylaxis symptoms.[17–19]

The diagnostic accuracy of SPT can vary based on the allergen, whether commercial extract or fresh foods are used, and amongst practices in how tests are performed and interpreted.[20] PTP testing has more test-to-test variability compared with commercial extract and is considered a less reliable and reproducible test. It is difficult to standardize the concentration of the food allergen with PTP testing, and fresh foods may be more likely to cause skin irritation resulting in false positives. For example, fish juice containing high molecular weight polypeptides is known to irritate the skin of fish mongers.[11] As such, a negative result can be more useful than a positive result. Generally, it is thought that the negative predictive value (NPV) of SPT can be quite high, especially when testing with fresh foods, such as fresh nuts, or nut flours when compared with commercial extracts. Testing for foods such as raw egg, milk, and wheat also has good NPV when skin test results are negative or measurably decrease over time.[21,22] For protein CU or PCD, clinical correlation is necessary to improve diagnostic utility of these tests.

Risks of SPT include systemic reaction, although this risk is minimal (0.07%); risk is increased when fresh foods are used for skin testing.[11,23] Cases described with PTP testing include development of dyspnea, angioedema, and circulatory collapse with testing with pine nuts; pruritus and urticaria with testing with raw and cooked fish and meat; bronchoconstriction with testing with roasted peanut; and severe anaphylaxis with fresh fruit testing.[12] Thus, SPT should be performed in an allergist's office that is equipped to handle anaphylactic reactions with injectable epinephrine available for immediate use. As such, patients with poorly controlled asthma, especially those with active wheezing, should not undergo SPT.

Alternative to SPT include measurement of specific IgE to the allergens in question, although both tests have low specificity.[24] IgE is quantified in kilounits per liter (kU/L) and measured using enzymatic immunoassays, which are usually automated, such as the ImmunoCAP system.[24] A negative cut-off of less than 0.35 kU/L is used, which has a high sensitivity but poor specificity to diagnose food allergy. The specificity of IgE testing can vary based on allergen, for example, wheat and soy IgE are poorly predictive for food allergy, and more useful tests when combined with clinical history.[24] For certain allergens, such as peanut, cut-offs have been determined for 95% positive predictive value, which for peanut is 15 kU/L, which has a specificity of 96.8% and sensitivity of 28.4% in one UK study.[25] IgE testing to allergen components or component-resolved diagnostics allows for measuring of IgE to a specific allergen, rather than a commercially prepared extract that contains multiple allergens. There are no studies in use of component-resolved diagnostics for diagnosis of PCD or CU; however, such studies are common in cases of oral allergy syndrome, which is a mechanistically similar disease.[26] Future investigations are needed to better understand the phenotypic differences in patients experiencing CU and PCD as distinct from patients experiencing anaphylaxis and why their disease process does not progress in severity, despite the presence of IgE. Possibly, the patients with CU have IgE directed to particular food proteins associated with cutaneous-only reactions.

## ADDITIONAL TESTING

Additional laboratory studies for the investigation of immediate food allergy include specific IgE/total IgE ratio, specific IgG4/IgE ratios, IgE to allergen peptides, and T-cell assays.[24] These have been used in clinical research but are not yet used in general allergy practice. Basophil activation tests (BAT) have shown promise, as they assess IgE functionality by measuring the ability of IgE to activate basophils after allergen stimulation.[24] Unlike traditional serum IgE testing, which measures an IgE level, BAT uses whole blood to measure IgE function, which depends on epitope specificity, affinity, and clonality.[24] BAT has improved specificity over IgE testing, while retaining sensitivity, and may be a useful test in patients who may have elevated total IgE levels, such as those with AD who may have high circulating specific IgE to foods of unclear clinical significance. BAT has been studied in oral allergy syndrome to identify culprit foods, indicating it may have use in CU and PCD as well.[24]

The gold standard for diagnosis of immediate IgE-mediated food allergy is double-blind placebo-controlled oral food challenge (OFC), although this is rarely performed in the clinical setting. Typically, open observed graded food challenges are performed, and the risk of the challenge will depend on the capabilities and comfort of the allergist practice. Challenges are performed based on the combined interpretation of clinical history, SPT results, and IgE levels, and when a diagnosis of food allergy is in question. Referrals to an allergist should be made for OFC to clear patients for ingestion of a food in the safest possible manner and may not exclude the presence of delayed food-related AD exacerbations. However, avoidance of foods based on food-related exacerbations can result in further sensitization and increase risk of anaphylaxis on reintroduction of a food after avoidance.[27] Thus, elimination diets are not typically recommended for delayed food-related AD exacerbations.

## GUIDELINES

In 2015, the Learning Early about Peanut (LEAP) trial published findings that were pivotal in changing guidelines for pediatricians and dermatologists alike on how to counsel patients on the prevention of food allergy. In high-risk patients with severe

AD and/or hen's egg allergy, early screening for peanut allergy subsequently followed by early peanut introduction successfully prevented the development of peanut allergy in a statistically significant number of patients when compared with an avoidance control.[28]

Severe AD was self-defined through parental questionnaire if one of the following criteria were met in the infant: (1) frequent need for treatment with topical corticosteroids or calcineurin inhibitors, (2) parental description of "a very bad rash in joints and creases or "a very bad itchy, dry, oozing, or crusted rash," or (3) a severe SCORing Atopic Dermatitis (SCORAD) grade ($\geq$40) by a clinician before or at the time of screening.[29] Egg allergy was defined as (1) SPT of greater than or equal to 6 mm with raw hen's egg white, the more allergenic portion of whole egg without history of egg tolerance, or (2) SPT greater than or equal to 3 mm with pasteurized hen's egg white with history of allergic reaction to egg. Using these definitions, in infants meeting these criteria, the prevalence of peanut allergy was 35.3% in the avoidance group and 10.6% in the consumption group ($P = .004$).[28] Thus, the LEAP findings resulted in formal guidelines from the National Institute of Allergy and Infectious Disease (NIAID) on early peanut introduction for clinicians, which suggest that infants in the high-risk categories with severe AD or hen's egg allergy undergo screening via SPT or peanut-specific IgE testing before peanut introduction.[30]

## FOOD ALLERGEN INTRODUCTION

Clinicians in family medicine, pediatrics, and dermatology are advised to use serum IgE testing to avoid delay in peanut introduction, based on negative results. This first-level screening and guidance by becomes even more important in a viral pandemic, as medical procedures, such as OFC, are not always feasible.[30] Infants with positive peanut IgE (IgE $\geq$0.35 kU/L) are to be referred to an allergist for SPT, and the allergist is then advised to perform supervised feeding or graded OFC for peanut SPT of 3 to 7 mm. Guidelines are unclear for SPT greater than 8 mm, but generally these patients are considered allergic and should be counseled to carry an epinephrine autoinjector and advised of the risks of accidental ingestion and cross-contamination. Infants with mild or moderate AD are advised to introduce 2 g of peanut protein (2 teaspoons of peanut butter) at home allowing for clinicians outside of allergy (nonallergists) to subsequently guide patients on allergenic food introductions. Once introduced, caregivers should aim to give the infant 6 to 7 g of peanut protein weekly (approximately 2 teaspoons of peanut butter 3 times weekly), which is an important step to help maintain tolerance.

Since the publication of these findings, similar studies have taken place, examining early introduction of other foods, such as cow's milk and hen's egg.[31,32] In the Enquiring About Tolerance (EAT) study, infants with moderate AD (SCORAD 15 to <40) developed less hen's egg allergy if introduced to the food early.[31] The Canadian Healthy Infant Longitudinal Development (CHILD) study data showed that early introduction is also an effective strategy in the general population, and both LEAP and the Health-Nuts study, an observational food allergy study in Australia, have shown that early introductions are generally safe with low rates of reaction (2%) that are primarily cutaneous in nature.[28,30,32,33] These studies demonstrate the safety and efficacy of early food introduction, and thus a recent consensus approach to introduction of allergenic foods suggests that all allergenic foods, not just peanut and egg can be introduced early and that screening for food allergies in infants prior to introduction is not required.[34] General food allergy prevalence in US children is estimated to be at least 8%, and increasing[35] In the 10 years from 1997 to 2007, food allergy prevalence increased 18% among US children.[36] This risk and increase is further amplified in children with AD, regardless of race or geography, with high rates of sensitization seen in African-American, Hispanic-American, and even South African children with AD.[37–39]

Because infants with AD are a subset prone to sensitization, presence of allergen-specific IgE may be clinically insignificant.[40,41] In a study of more than 1000 infants with mild-to-severe AD treated with 1% pimecrolimus cream, and no prior history of food allergy, allergen-specific IgE decision points (14 kU/L for peanut, 15 kU/L for cow's milk, and 7 kU/L for egg white) poorly predicted the development of food allergy based on clinical history. However, OFCs were not performed in this study, and the investigators emphasize that OFC is "the only definitive test for food allergy." In addition, infants of all AD severity were screened in this study, whereas NIAID guidelines suggest screening only those with severe eczema, defined as persistent or recurring typical rash requiring frequent topical prescription treatment.[30,40] For patients with mild-to-moderate AD, referral to the allergist is not necessary to guide food introductions, and they can make recommendations for feeding at home per guidelines. Because of the risk of cutaneous sensitization, feeding practice guidelines have recommended barrier ointment application before the feed and giving feeds with a long spoon to avoid skin exposure.[42] If local reactions such as eczema flares of the cheeks are observed, these can be managed with skincare, and further referral should be made for signs of immediate hypersensitivity, such as urticaria, respiratory difficulty, throat symptoms, or vomiting.

## SUMMARY

Infants with AD are at risk for the development of FA, and this risk increases with increasing severity of AD.[34,40] Early introduction of foods has been identified as a strategy for prevention of food allergy in infants, and does not require routine screening, particularly in those with milder AD.[34] Reassurance of parents on the safety of home introductions is important, as allergen avoidance due to worry or anxiety may result in delayed introduction and development of food allergy.[34] Referral to an allergist may be considered to guide introduction of allergens, such as peanut to infants with severe AD, who are at higher risk for development of food allergy. Infants with mild-to-moderate AD can be counseled to begin allergenic foods introduction at 6 months of life, and once introduced it is important to encourage regular consumption to maintain tolerance. Food-related AD exacerbations do not warrant allergist referral and can often be managed with skincare. To minimize the development of food allergy in at-risk infants with severe AD, screening with SPT or IgE may be appropriate. Screening by clinicians in family medicine, dermatology, and pediatrics would be through serum IgE testing, and any positive result would warrant referral to an allergist, who is pivotal in determining the relevance of these tests.[41] Allergists may screen patients using SPT and IgE testing and consider OFC for any positive IgE or SPT between 3 to 7 mm. Referral to the allergist (see **Box 1**) is also appropriate in instances of PCD or CU for SPT to determine the causative allergen, if patients have associated atopic disease or whenever food allergy is suspected based on clinical history.

## CLINICS CARE POINTS

- Dermatologic disorders, such as atopic dermatitis, contact urticaria, and protein contact dermatitis may place a patient at risk for development of systemic food allergy.
- The risk for food allergy increases with increasing severity of atopic dermatitis.
- Routine screening of food allergy is not recommended.

- Early introduction of allergenic foods may be protective against the development of food allergy.
- Screening may be warranted in high risk infants for foods, such as peanut and hen's egg.

## DISCLOSURE

The author has nothing to disclose.

## REFERENCES

1. Roerdink EM, Flokstra-de Blok BMJ, Blok JL, et al. Association of food allergy and atopic dermatitis exacerbations. Ann Allergy Asthma Immunol 2016;116:334–8.
2. Bergmann MM, Caubet JC, Boguniewicz M, et al. Evaluation of food allergy in patients with atopic dermatitis. J Allergy Clin Immunol Pract 2013;1(1):22–8.
3. Kim BS, Wang K, Siracusa MC, et al. Basophils promote innate lymphoid cell responses in inflamed skin. J Immunol 2014;193:3717–25.
4. Leung DYM, Calatroni A, Zaramela LS, et al. The nonlesional skin surface distinguishes atopic dermatitis with food allergy as a unique endotype. Sci Transl Med 2019;11(480):eaav2685.
5. Tordesillas L, Goswami R, Benede S, et al. Skin exposure promotes a Th2-dependent sensitization to peanut allergens. J Clin Immunol 2014;124(11):4965–75.
6. Noti M, Kim BS, Siracusa MC, et al. Exposure to food allergens through inflamed skin promotes intestinal food allergy through the thymic stromal lymphopoietin–basophil axis. J Allergy Clin Immunol 2014;133(5):1390–9.
7. Fukuie T, Yasuoka R, Fujiyama T, et al. Palmar hyperlinearity in early childhood atopic dermatitis is associated with filaggrin mutation and sensitization to egg. Pediatr Dermatol 2019;36(2):213–8.
8. Brar KK, Calatroni A, Berdyshev E, et al. Hyperlinear palms as a clinical finding in peanut allergy. J Allergy Clin Immunol Pract 2020;8(8):2823–5.
9. Barbaud A, Poreaux C, Penven E, et al. Occupational protein contact dermatitis. Eur J Dermatol 2015;25(6):527–34.
10. Helaskoski E, Suojalehto H, Kuuliala O, et al. Occupational contact urticaria and protein contact dermatitis: causes and concomitant airway diseases. Contact Dermatitis 2017;77(6):390–6.
11. Anagnostou A. Con: skin prick testing with fresh foods. Ann Allergy Asthma Immunol 2020;124:443–4.
12. Nelson H, Knoetzer J, Bucher B. Effect of distance between sites and region of the body on results of skin prick tests. J Allergy Clin Immunol 1996;97(2):596–601.
13. Raith M, Klug C, Sesztak-Greinecker G, et al. Unusual sensitization to parvalbumins from certain fish species. Ann Allergy Asthma Immunol 2014;113:571–8.
14. Vlieg-Boerstra BJ, van de Weg WE. Where to prick the apple for skin testing? Allergy 2013;68:1196–8.
15. Turner PJ, Gray PEA, Wong M. Anaphylaxis to apple and orange seed. J Allergy Clin Immunol 2011;128(6):1363–5.
16. Rodrigues-Alves R, Lopez A, Pereira-Santos MC, et al. Clinical, anamnestic and serological features of peach allergy in Portugal. Int Arch Allergy Immunol 2009;149(1):65–73.

17. Ando Y, Miyamoto M, Kato M, et al. Pru p 7 Predicts Severe reactions after ingestion of peach in Japanese children and adolescents. Int Arch Allergy Immunol 2020;181(3):183–90.

18. Klingebiel C, Chantran Y, Arif-Lusson R, et al. Pru p 7 sensitization is a predominant cause of severe, cypress pollen-associated peach allergy. Clin Exp Allergy 2019;49(4):526–36.

19. Asero R, Antonicelli L, Arena A, et al. Causes of food-induced anaphylaxis in Italian adults: a multi-centre study. Int Arch Allergy Immunol 2009;150(3):271–7.

20. Oppenheimer J, Nelson H. Skin testing a survey of allergists. Ann Allergy Asthma Immunol 2006;96:19–23.

21. Elizur A, Goldberg MR. Pro: Skin prick testing with fresh foods. Ann Allergy Asthma Immunol 2020;124:441–2.

22. Uncuoglu A, Simsek IE, Cogurlu MT, et al. Utility of fresh egg skin prick test and egg yolk specific immunoglobulin E for outgrowth. Ann Allergy Asthma Immunol 2020;125:418–24.

23. Sellaturay P, Nasser S, Ewan P. The incidence and features of systemic reactions to skin prick tests. Ann Allergy Asthma Immunol 2015;115:229–33.

24. Santos AF, Brough HA. Making the most of in vitro tests to diagnose food allergy. J Allergy Clin Immunol 2017;5(2):237–48.

25. Roberts G, Lack G. Diagnosing peanut allergy with skin prick and specific IgE testing. J Allergy Clin Immunol 2005;115:1291–6.

26. McFadden J. Immunologic contact urticaria. Immunol Allergy Clin N Am 2014;34: 157–67.

27. Change A, Robinson R, Cai M, et al. Natural history of food triggered atopic dermatitis and development of immediate reactions in children. J Allergy Clin Immunol Pract 2016;4(2):229–36.

28. Du Toit G, Roberts G, Sayre PH, et al. Randomized trial of peanut consumption in infants at risk for peanut allergy. N Engl J Med 2015;372:803–13.

29. Du Toit G, Roberts G, Sayre PH, et al. Identifying infants at high risk of peanut allergy: the Learning Early About Peanut Allergy (LEAP) screening study. J Allergy Clin Immunol 2013;131:135–43.

30. Togias A, Cooper SF, Acebal ML, et al. Addendum guidelines for the prevention of peanut allergy in the United States: report of the National Institute of Allergy and Infectious Diseases-sponsored expert panel. J Allergy Clin Immunol 2017; 139:29–44.

31. Perkin MR, Logan K, Marrs T, et al. Enquiring About Tolerance (EAT) study: feasibility of an early allergenic food introduction regimen. J Allergy Clin Immunol 2016;137(5):1477–86.e8.

32. Simons E, Balshaw R, Lefebvre DL, et al. Timing of introduction, sensitization, and allergy to highly allergenic foods at age 3 years in a general-population Canadian cohort. J Allergy Clin Immunol Pract 2020;8(1):166–75.e10.

33. Osborne NJ, Koplin JJ, Martin PE, et al. The HealthNuts population-based study of paediatric food allergy: validity, safety and acceptability. Clin Exp Allergy 2010; 40(10):1516–22.

34. Fleischer DM, Chan ES, et al. A Consensus Approach to the Primary Prevention of Food Allergy through Nutrition: Guidance from the American Academy of Allergy, Asthma, and Immunology; American College of Allergy, Asthma, and Immunology; and the Canadian Society for Allergy and Clinical Immunology. J Allergy Clin Immunol Pract 2021;9(1):22–43.

35. Gupta RS, Springston EE, Warrier MR, et al. The prevalence, severity, and distribution of childhood food allergy in the United States. Pediatrics 2011;128(1): e9–17.

36. Branum AM, Lukacs SL. Food allergy among children in the United States. Pediatrics 2009;124:1549–55.

37. Gray CL, Levin ME, Zar HJ, et al. Food allergy in South African children with atopic dermatitis. Pediatr Allergy Immunol 2016;27:709–15.

38. Gray CL, Levin ME, du Toit G. Egg sensitization, allergy and component patterns in African children with atopic dermatitis. Pediatr Allergy Immunol 2016;27: 709–15.

39. Mahdavinia M, Fox SR, Smith BM, et al. Racial differences in food allergy phenotype and health care utilization among US children. J Allergy Clin Immunol Pract 2017;5(2):352–7.

40. Spergel JM, Boguniewicz M, Schneider L, et al. Food allergy in infants with atopic dermatitis: limitations of food-specific IgE measurements. Pediatrics 2015;136(6): e1530–8.

41. Robinson RG, Singh AM. Controversies in allergy: food testing and dietary avoidance in atopic dermatitis. J Allergy Clin Immunol Pract 2019;7(1):35–9.

42. Nedorost ST, Raffi J, Brar KK, et al. Art of prevention: the importance of feeding traditions. Int J Womens Dermatol 2019;5:378–80.

# Moving?

## Make sure your subscription moves with you!

To notify us of your new address, find your **Clinics Account Number** (located on your mailing label above your name), and contact customer service at:

**Email: journalscustomerservice-usa@elsevier.com**

**800-654-2452** (subscribers in the U.S. & Canada)
**314-447-8871** (subscribers outside of the U.S. & Canada)

**Fax number: 314-447-8029**

**Elsevier Health Sciences Division
Subscription Customer Service
3251 Riverport Lane
Maryland Heights, MO 63043**

*To ensure uninterrupted delivery of your subscription, please notify us at least 4 weeks in advance of move.

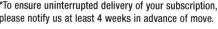
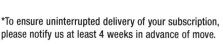